AF335592

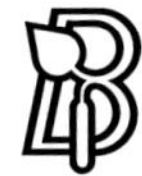

Milestones in Drug Therapy
MDT

Series Editors

Prof. Dr. Michael J. Parnham
PLIVA
Research Institute
Prilaz baruna Filipovica 25
10000 Zagreb
Croatia

Prof. Dr. J. Bruinvels
INFARM
Sweelincklaan 75
NL-3723 JC Bilthoven
The Netherlands

Anxiolytics

Edited by M. Briley and D. Nutt

Birkhäuser Verlag
Basel . Boston . Berlin

Editors

Dr. Mike Briley
Institut de Recherche Pierre Fabre
Parc Industriel de la Chartreuse
81100 Castres
France

Professor David Nutt
University of Bristol
Psychopharmacology Unit
School of Medical Science
University Walk
Bristol BS8 1TD
UK

Library of Congress Cataloging-in-Publication Data

Anxiolytics / edited by M. Briley and D. Nutt,
    p. cm — Milestones in drug therapy)
  Includes bibliographical references and index.
  ISBN 3764360321 (alk. paper)
  I. Tranquilizing drugs. I. Briley, M. II. Nutt, David J., 1951- III. Series.

  RM333 A582 2000
  615'.7882–dc21   00-033748

Deutsche Bibliothek Cataloging-in-Publication Data

Anxiolytics / ed. by M. Briley and D. Nutt. - Basel ; Boston ; Berlin : Birkhäuser, 2000
  (Milestones in drug therapy)
  ISBN 3-7643-6032-1

ISBN 3-7643-6032-1 Birkhäuser Verlag, Basel - Boston - Berlin

Contents

List of contributors

Spilios V. Argyropoulos, Psychopharmacology Unit, School of Medical Sciences, University Walk, Bristol BS8 1TD, England; e-mail: spilios.argyropoulos@bristol.ac.uk

David S. Baldwin, Senior Lecturer in Psychiatry, Mental Health Group, Faculty of Medicine, Health and Biological Sciences, University of Southampton, UK; University Department of Psychiatry, Royal South Hants Hospital, Brintons Terrace, Southampton, UK; e-mail: dsb1@soton.ac.uk

Jon Birtwistle, Training Fellow, Primary Medical Care Group, Faculty of Medicine, Health and Biological Sciences, University of Southampton, UK; e-mail: jb11@soton.ac.uk

Michael Bös, Boehringer Ingelheim, Virology Research Center, Montreal, Canada

Raimund Buller, Quintiles, 3–5, rue Maurice Ravel, F-92594 Levallois-Perret, France; e-mail: raimund.buller@quintiles.com

Graham D. Burrows, Department of Psychiatry, University of Melbourne, Austin & Repatriation Medical Centre, Heidelberg 3084, Victoria, Australia

Guy Griebel, Sanofi-Synthelabo, 31 avenue Paul Vaillant-Couturier, 92220 Bagneux, France; e-mail: guy.griebel@sanofi.synthelabo.com

Rudolf Hoehn-Saric, 115 Meyer Building, Johns Hopkins Hospital, Baltimore, MD 21287-7115, USA; e-mail: rhoehn@welchlink.welch.jhu.edu

François Jenck, Roche Pharma Division, Preclinical CNS Research, CH-4070 Basel, Switzerland; e-mail: francois.jenck@roche.com

Karin M. Jorga, F. Hoffmann-La Roche, Dept. of Clinical Pharmacology, Grenzachstrasse 124, CH-4070 Basel, Switzerland; e-mail: karin.jorga@roche.com

Louise R. Levine, Lilly Research Laboratories, Eli Lilly and Company, Lilly Corporate Center DC 1730, Indianapolis, IN 46285, USA; e-mail: lulu@lilly.com

Caroline McGrath, Department of Psychiatry, University of Melbourne, Austin & Repatriation Medical Centre, Heidelberg 3084, Victoria, Australia; e-mail: c.mcgrath@medicine.unimelb.edu.au

James R. Martin, F. Hoffmann-La Roche, Preclinical CNS Research, Grenzachstrasse 124, CH-4070 Basel, Switzerland

Jean-Luc Moreau, F. Hoffmann-La Roche, Preclinical CNS Research, Grenzachstrasse 124, CH-4070 Basel, Switzerland

Chantal Moret, Les Grèzes, La Verdarié, 81100 Castres, France; e-mail: chantal.moret@neurobiz.com

Trevor R. Norman, Department of Psychiatry, University of Melbourne, Austin

& Repatriation Medical Centre, Heidelberg 3084, Victoria, Australia; e-mail: trevor@austin.unimelb.edu.au

David J. Nutt, Psychopharmacology Unit, School of Medical Sciences, University Walk, Bristol BS8 1TD, England; e-mail: David.J.Nutt@bristol.ac.uk

Ghislaine Perrault, Sanofi-Synthelabo, 31 avenue Paul Vaillant-Couturier, 92220 Bagneux, France

William Z. Potter, Lilly Research Laboratories, Eli Lilly and Company, Lilly Corporate Center DC 1730, Indianapolis, IN 46285, USA; e-mail: wzp@lilly.com

David J. Sanger, Sanofi-Synthelabo, 31 avenue Paul Vaillant-Couturier, 92220 Bagneux, France

Darius K. Shayegan, Clinical Neuroscience Research Center, 8899 University Center Lane, Suite 130, San Diego, California 92122, USA

Phil Skolnick, Neuroscience Discovery, Lilly Research Laboratories, Lilly Corporate Center, Drop Code 0510, Indianapolis, IN 46285, USA; e-mail: SKOLNICK_PHIL@LILLY.COM

Heinz Stadler, F. Hoffmann-La Roche, Preclinical CNS Research, Grenzachstrasse 124, CH-4070 Basel, Switzerland

Stephen M. Stahl, Department of Psychiatry, University of California, San Diego, USA

Jürgen Wichmann, F. Hoffmann-La Roche, Preclinical CNS Research, Grenzachstrasse 124, CH-4070 Basel, Switzerland

Preface

For over thirty years the benzodiazepines monopolised not only the anxiolytic market but also clinical and animal research in anxiety. Indeed many animal tests developed since the 1960s have been optimised for the benzodiazepines and some programmes have even screened candidates as potential anxiolytics on their benzodiazepine-like side-effects rather than their anxiolytic activity. With the realisation of the drawbacks of the benzodiazepines, namely their potential for tolerance and dependency, there has been a renewed interest in alternative anxiolytics both from existing drugs such as the tricyclic and monoamine oxidase antidepressants and from newer agents such as buspirone. In addition anxiety is no longer considered to be a unique entity but rather an umbrella term for a series of specific anxiety disorders such as panic disorder without or with agoraphobia, generalised anxiety disorder (GAD), specific phobias, social phobias and post-traumatic stress disorder (PTSD). These new clinical categories have opened another dimension in the therapy of anxiety requiring the optimisation of treatments for different syndromes.

This book is a critical review of today's anxiolytics and those that may become the anxiolytics of tomorrow. What is clear is that currently there are few clinically satisfactory alternatives to the benzodiazepines for the treatment of acute anxiety. For chronic anxiety, it is generally agreed that benzodiazepines are not the treatment of first choice. The tricyclic and monoamine oxidase antidepressants, the serotonin reuptake inhibitors and buspirone offer better solutions for chronic anxiety but they are still far from being ideal.

The challenge for tomorrow is not only to find more efficacious treatments with a more rapid onset of action and an acceptable side-effect profile but to define more precisely which agents may treat the different anxiety disorders. Serotonin is a major target, particularly through the 5-HT1A, 5-HT1B and 5-HT2 receptors. The amino acid receptors, the glutamate complex in particular, is being intensively investigated as a potential target for anxiolytics. Finally the involvement of a number of neuropeptides in the control of stress and anxious reactions is becoming increasingly clear and new chemical agents are being developed to probe these potential anxiolytic targets.

This intense research activity suggests that we may soon have a whole new range of options for the treatment of anxiety disorders and so be able to finally leave behind us "the age of anxiety".

Mike Briley
David Nutt

Anxiolytics
ed. by M. Briley and D. Nutt
© 2000 Birkhäuser Verlag/Switzerland

The benzodiazepines: a brief review of pharmacology and therapeutics

Caroline McGrath, Graham D. Burrows and Trevor R. Norman

Department of Psychiatry, University of Melbourne, Austin & Repatriation Medical Centre, Heidelberg 3084, Victoria, Australia

Introduction

Benzodiazepines were first discovered in the mid 1950s when Sternbach, a medicinal chemist in New Jersey, began synthesising compounds with a bicyclic nucleus benzo-1, 4-diazepine structure. One compound, chlordiazepoxide (Fig. 1), exhibited sedative, anticonvulsant and muscle relaxant properties, which were confirmed by clinical studies and was launched as an anxiolytic in 1960 under the trade name Librium. A second compound, diazepam (valium), which was more potent and had a broader spectrum of activity than chlordiazepoxide [1], was introduced in 1963. Since then, numerous analogues of the benzodiazepine structure have been developed and introduced into clinical practice.

Following their introduction, benzodiazepines were generally regarded as a safe and effective alternative to their predecessors, the barbiturates, which had by this time been recognised as having a high abuse potential [2]. However, by the 1970s and the 1980s opinions began to change regarding the use of the

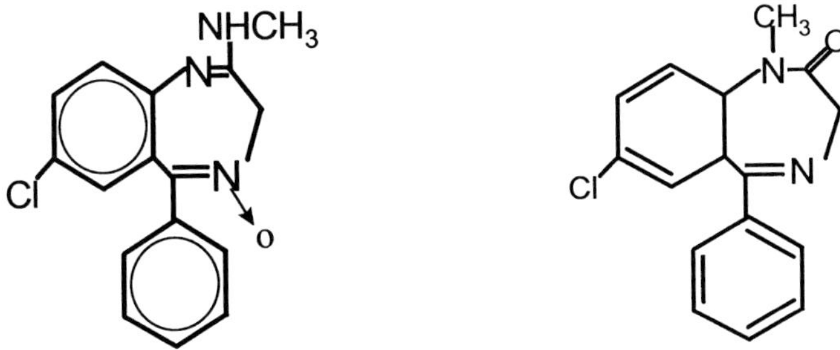

1.1 **Chlordiazepoxide**   *1.2* **Diazepam**

Figure 1. (1) Chlordiazepoxide, (2) Diazepam.

benzodiazepines as questions were raised about their unwanted side-effects and possible dependence properties. As a consequence, in 1986, Schedule 4 of the Misuse of Drugs Act (UK) was introduced to control the prescribing of the benzodiazepines (cited in [2]).

Mechanism of action

In the mid 1970s attempts to elucidate the mechanism of action of these compounds noted the requirement for the presence of gamma-aminobutyric acid (GABA) in order to exert their effects. Subsequently, high affinity binding sites (benzodiazepine receptors (BZR)) identified in the central nervous system (CNS) [3, 4] were reported to be the site of action of these compounds. BZRs have since been identified in the periphery (i.e. benzodiazepine-3 receptors, abundant in the kidney) as well as the CNS and are referred to as peripheral and central BZRs respectively.

GABA is an inhibitory neurotransmitter and is one of the most widely distributed neurotransmitters in the mammalian brain [5], in fact it has been reported to act at 40% of synapses in the brain [5]. GABA acts on two classes of GABAergic receptors namely, $GABA_A$ and $GABA_B$ receptors. The $GABA_A$ receptor has been shown to be closely associated with the benzodiazepine binding site in the CNS. $GABA_A$ receptors in the brain are coupled to chloride ion channels. When GABA is released into the synaptic cleft it activates the $GABA_A$ receptor, resulting in the opening of the chloride ion channel, and an influx of ions into the cell. On their own, benzodiazepines exert little effect on the ion channel, however the presence of GABA enhances the effect of benzodiazepines on the chloride ion channels. Unlike the barbiturates, which increase the frequency of channel opening, the benzodiazepines exert their

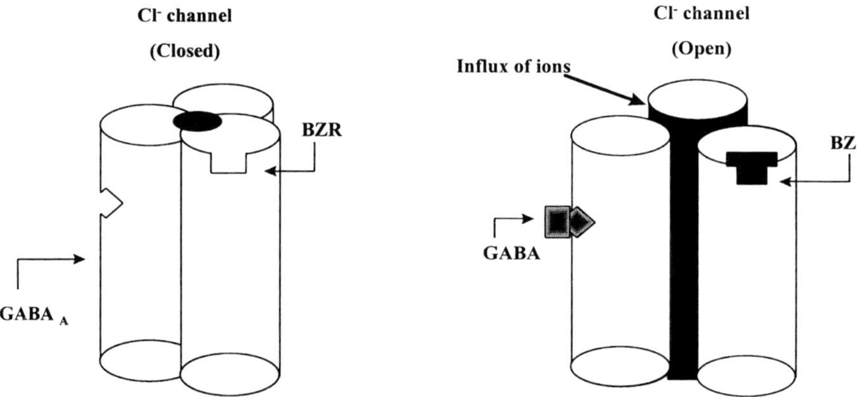

Figure 2. Model of the mechanism of action of the benzodiazepines.

effects on chloride ion channels by increasing the duration of channel opening [6]. It is this state of hyperpolarisation that is believed to mediate the anxiolytic effects of the benzodiazepines [7].

Since its discovery, various categories of ligands have been identified which act at the benzodiazepine receptor complex [8], namely, agonists (which include the benzodiazepines), antagonists (such as flumazenil, which unlike the benzodiazepines have relatively little effect on GABAergic transmission and block their actions) and inverse agonists, which exert the opposite effects to the benzodiazepines, thus increasing anxiety [8]. Furthermore, the existence of the BZR complex has led to the suggestion of the existence of an endogenous compound in the body which may act as a "natural anxiolytic". Numerous substances have been proposed including the β carbolines. There is evidence that some members of this class may act as anxiogenic agents in man, while others may exhibit similar effects to those elicited by the benzodiazepines, thus reducing anxiety and preventing convulsions. Another compound that has been investigated is the polypeptide, diazepam binding inhibitor (DBI) which exhibits inverse agonist activity [8]. Studies have shown that DBI has anxiogenic properties and it has been reported to block benzodiazepine receptors in the brain under certain conditions [5].

Pharmacokinetics

Large differences exist in the pharmacokinetic parameters of the various benzodiazepines [9], which have been classified according to their various elimination half-lives (t1/2). Diazepam for example, has a long t1/2 of 20–90 h, while the t1/2 of midazolam is approximately 1–3 h (Tab. 1). Such differences in the rate of elimination may influence the choice of drug for a particular indication [10]. For drugs with a short elimination half-life, accumulation on chronic dosing is minimal, since the first dose of the drug is generally eliminated before the second dose is administered [11]. As hypnotics, benzodiazepines with a short elimination half-life, such as midazolam and triazolam may be the drugs of choice, since the therapeutic effect of the drug should be restricted to the night [9]. For anxiety however, benzodiazepines with a long elimination half-life may be more effective since a prolonged therapeutic effect is required [9, 12]. Elimination half-life however is not the only determinant of duration of drug action. Other factors such as lipophilicity (and therefore distribution of the drug), absorption rate and the presence or absence of active metabolites are also important [13]. In fact it has been suggested that the most important pharmacokinetic variable for determining duration of drug action following single dosing is the extent of drug distribution [14]. Diazepam for example, which has a long t1/2 (35 to 50 h), is highly lipophilic and as such has a wide volume of distribution, so plasma and brain concentrations, necessary for therapeutic effect, are not maintained over an extended period of time [11]. The intermediate acting benzodiazepine, lorazepam (12 to 20 h) on the

Table 1. Pharmacokinetic properties of the benzodiazepines

Drug	Mean t1/2 (h)	Ref.	Main metabolite(s)	Active
Chlordiazepoxide	8–28	26	desmethyldiazepam	+
			demoxepam	+
Diazepam	35–50	46	desmethyldiazepam	+
Temazepam	5–8		oxazepam	+
Flurazepam	1–2	38	N-Desalkylflurazepam	+
Nitrazepam	16–40		–	
Oxazepam	6–28		–	
Lorazepam	13–17		–	
Loprazolam	10–16	16	–	
Clorazepate	2.4	50	desmethyldiazepam	+
Lormetazepam	8–12		–	
Flunitrazepam	9–25	14	desmethylflunitrazepam	+
Alprazolam	12	12	β-hydroxy alprazolam	–
			4-hydroxy alprazolam	–
Triazolam	1.8–5.9	17	7α-hydroxytriazolam	+
Midazolam	1.5–3	18	α-hydroxymidazolam	+

other hand, is less extensively distributed, and as such may have a longer duration of action since effective plasma concentrations are maintained longer [11].

The presence of active metabolites is also a distinguishing factor between the benzodiazepines [15]. Long half-life benzodiazepines such as diazepam and flurazepam, generally give rise to active metabolites [16] which may prolong the activity of the drug. Intermediate- or short-acting benzodiazepines on the other hand either have few active metabolites [16], or have active metabolites which lack sufficient potency at the receptor to produce a therapeutic effect. Alprazolam is metabolised to α-hydroxyalprazolam and 4-hydroxyalprazolam (Fig. 3) [17], and although α-hydroxyalprazolam has pharmacological activity [18] its low receptor affinity and low plasma concentration (less than 10% of alprazolam) suggest that it is unlikely to contribute to the therapeutic effect of alprazolam [19].

Three main pathways have been identified for the metabolism of the benzodiazepines [19], each sensitive to and controlled by different factors [11]. Alprazolam for example is metabolised by oxidation, which is sensitive to differences in population characteristics and disease state. Greenblatt and Wright, [18] reported that alprazolam clearance is greatly reduced in the elderly and in patients with cirrhosis. Similar effects have been reported for the metabolism of midazolam [20, 21]. Age-related effects on clearance of benzodiazepines which undergo metabolism by glucuronidation (oxazepam, lorazepam and temazepam) or nitroreduction (nitrazepam and clonazepam) appear to be minimal [19, 22, 23] suggesting that these benzodiazepines may be safer for use in such populations, however this has yet to be validated [23].

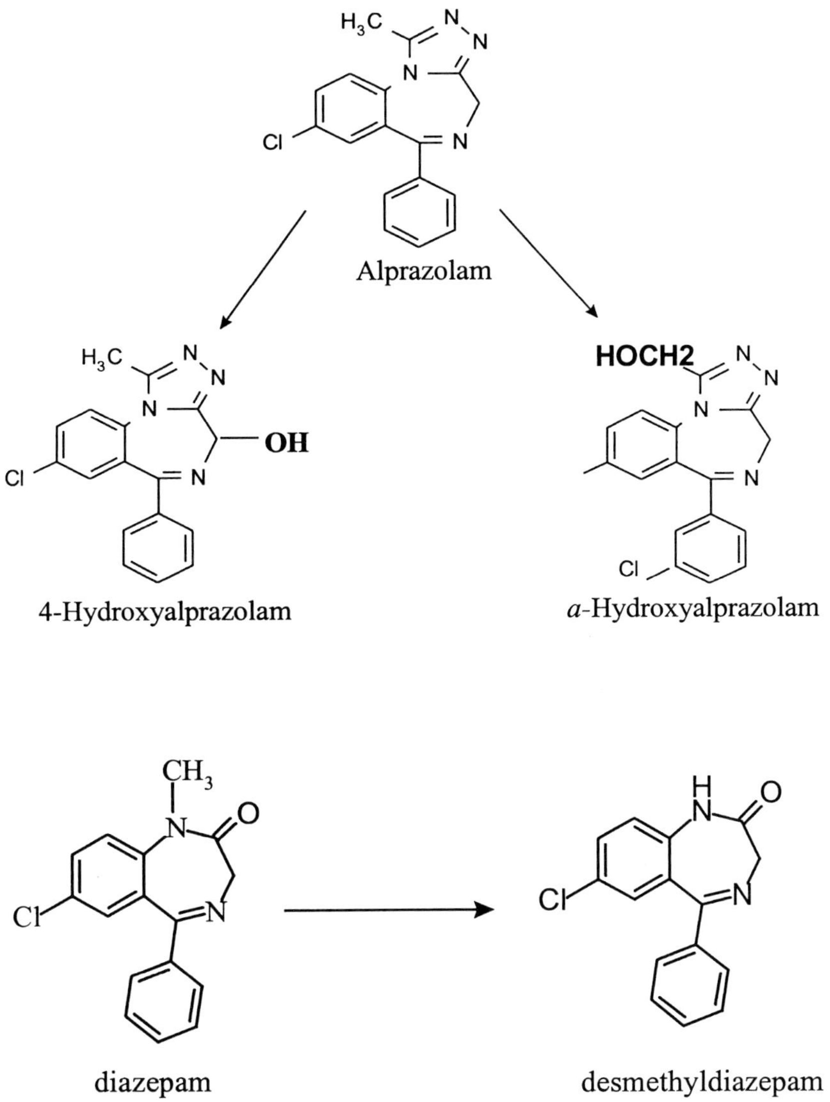

Figure 3. Alprazolam and Diazepam and their major metabolites.

Drug interactions

Since benzodiazepines are metabolised by the cytochrome P450 enzyme system the potential for drug interactions exists. Although more than 30 human CYP P450 enzymes have been identified most information available is about CYP 2D6, CYP 3A4 and CYP 1A2 [24], with CYP 2D6 and CYP 3A4 reported to account for approximately 90% of drug metabolism [19]. There is a potential therefore for both dangerous and beneficial drug interactions through induction or inhibition of these CYP enzymes [25]. Interactions between the benzodiazepines and other drugs have been reported with inhibitors of CYP 3A4 such as ketoconazole [26], cimetidine [27], and erythromycin [28, 29] which impair the metabolism of benzodiazepines, while inducers of this system increase their metabolism. Furukori et al. [30] found that carbamazepine, an inducer of CYP 3A4 increased the metabolism of alprazolam. Similar findings have been reported with rifampin [31] and phenytoin [32].

While the potential for drug interactions exists, most are of limited clinical significance but some important ones do occur [11]. Interactions have also been reported with the antipsychotic clozapine [34] and the antidepressants fluoxetine [35] and fluvoxamine [36]. The combination of a benzodiazepine and an antidepressant is frequently used in clinical practice with a potential for over-sedation due to a pharmacokinetic drug–drug interaction.

Increased knowledge of the cytochrome P450 systems, their inhibitors, inducers and substrates may help to avoid pharmacokinetic drug interactions [37] and as such improve patient treatment. Alcohol has been reported to increase the sedative effects of the benzodiazepines thus increasing psychomotor impairment [33] and reducing the ability to drive or operate machinery. This interaction probably represents a pharmacodynamic effect as both ethanol and benzodiazepines bind to the GABA–benzodiazepine complex. Alcohol is best avoided during benzodiazepine treatment.

Clinical use

Benzodiazepines are the most widely prescribed drugs in the treatment of anxiety disorders, showing efficacy in Generalised Anxiety Disorder, specific phobias and Panic Disorder, although antidepressants are usually the treatment of choice for Panic Disorder [11]. There is some evidence for their use in the treatment of social phobia [38–41] and obsessive compulsive disorder (OCD) [42, 43] however their efficacy for the treatment of post-traumatic stress disorder (PTSD) is less convincing [45, 66]. While benzodiazepines are effective for the acute treatment of anxiety, whether or not they maintain their anxiolytic properties on chronic administration remains unclear [11]. Some studies have reported beneficial effects of the benzodiazepines following long-term treatment, however others have failed to find therapeutic effects [45].

In addition to their anxiolytic properties, benzodiazepines exhibit anticonvulsant, sedative/hypnotic and muscle relaxant effects [46] and as such have indications for the treatment of anxiety, sleep disorders, *status epilepticus* and for prophylaxis in epilepsy [47]. There is some evidence for their use as adjunctive agents in the treatment of mania and acute psychosis, where they are generally combined with mood stabilisers and antipsychotics [48–51]. They are also first line therapy for the treatment of alcohol withdrawal

[52–53]. Benzodiazepines have shown some efficacy in the treatment of depression [54–55] possibly reflecting alleviation of secondary depressive symptoms such as anxiety and sleep disturbances, rather than a true antidepressant effect [56].

Side-effects

The clinical use of benzodiazepines is associated with a number of side-effects, which usually occur soon after administration or an increase in the dose. Generally side-effects are well tolerated with chronic treatment. One of the most commonly reported side-effects is day time sedation which is particularly evident following the administration of benzodiazepines with long elimination half-lives. In addition, most benzodiazepines appear to produce some level of psychomotor impairment, with deficits on general vigilance and divided attention tasks [57–59] reported. Performance on everyday tasks such as driving a car is impaired following benzodiazepine administration, particularly when given in high single doses or when combined with alcohol [60]. Deficits in the acquisition of new information have been noted and in some cases this may be impaired by as much as 66% [61, 62]. The duration of these effects can range from 3.5 h to 24 h depending on the benzodiazepine used [60], the dose administered, the sensitivity of the cognitive tests [62], the age of the individual and concomitant drug use [63]. Patients taking benzodiazepines are often unaware of their memory impairment, possibly because the problems are often quite subtle [63] and in fact may underestimate the benzodiazepine induced memory deficits [64]. While most benzodiazepines will produce some form of cognitive impairment it is more likely to occur with benzodiazepines that have a high affinity for benzodiazepine receptors or that are eliminated slowly or accumulate in the body [65]. It is important that patients are made aware of these potential side-effects of the benzodiazepines at the onset of treatment.

Other adverse events reported with benzodiazepine use include the development of aggressive behaviour, the "rage reaction". Although these reactions are relatively rare there have been numerous reports of violence and aggression associated with the use of these agents [46, 67–70]. No characteristics have been found which will help identify individuals susceptible to these reactions, it has been suggested that they occur more commonly in younger patients, although the elderly may also be at risk [71].

Other potential side-effects of benzodiazepines include drowsiness, fatigue, weakness, light headedness, ataxia, respiratory suppression, depression as well as physical dependence and withdrawal. Rebound anxiety or insomnia has been reported following discontinuation of both anxiolytic and hypnotic benzodiazepines even at therapeutic doses [60] and appears to vary from a "short lived" rebound anxiety/insomnia starting 1–4 days after the cessation of the benzodiazepines to a "full blown" rebound syndrome lasting 10 to 14 days [2,

72]. The dose and t1/2 of the benzodiazepine used and the personality characteristics of the individual patient appear to be associated with the development of withdrawal [2, 72, 73].

Attempts to develop novel anxiolytic agents with a reduced side-effect profile than currently available benzodiazepines have addressed the role of benzodiazepine partial agonists such as abercarnil, bretazenil and alpidem in anxiety. These agents have shown promising results in both preclinical [74] and clinical studies [75–77] and appear to have a reduced side-effect profile and decreased risk of dependence/withdrawal [78] than the benzodiazepines. Whether they will be more effective and useful anxiolytic agents than the benzodiazepines requires further investigation.

Conclusions

The benzodiazepines remain useful agents for the treatment of various anxiety disorders. The growing concern over withdrawal reactions on discontinuation has limited their use in recent years. Nevertheless the drugs provide rapid relief from anxiety, an advantage over most other agents used in the treatment of these conditions. It would seem unlikely that there are major advances to be made in the coming years with respect to therapeutics with this class of psychotropic agent. On the other hand, a better understanding of the mechanism of action of the benzodiazepines has been fundamental in developing the neurobiological basis of anxiety. Further developments in this area and in particular, the elucidation of the role of the subunits of the receptor, should provide further insights into the nature of different anxiety states. It could be expected that this increased knowledge would also lead to better therapeutic options, such as the development of drugs with specific anxiolytic actions lacking the side-effects of current agents. To some extent this has been achieved with the partial agonists, which have arisen due to expanded knowledge of the GABA$_A$ benzodiazepine receptor complex.

References

1 Sternbach LH (1983) The Discovery of CNS active 1,4-benzodiazepines. *In*: E Costa (ed.): *The benzodiazepines: from molecular biology to clinical practice*. Raven Press, New York, 1–6

2 Robertson JR, Treasure W (1996) Benzodiazepine abuse: nature and extent of the problem. *CNS Drugs* 5: 137–146

3 Braestrup C, Squires RF (1977) Specific benzodiazepine receptors in rat brain characterized by high-affinity (3H) diazepam binding. *Proc Natl Acad Sci USA* 74: 3805–3809

4 Mohler H, Okada T (1977) Benzodiazepine receptor: demonstration in the central nervous system. *Science* 198: 849–851

5 Leonard B (1992) *Fundamentals of psychopharmacology*. Chichester, John Wiley, 31

6 Study RE, Barker JL (1982) Cellular mechanisms of benzodiazepine actions. *JAMA* 247: 2147–2151

7 Breier A, Paul SM (1988) Anxiety and the benzodiazepine – GABA receptor complex. *In*: M Roth,

R Noyes, GD Burrows (eds): *Handbook of anxiety*. Elsevier Science Publishers, Amsterdam, 193–212

8 Pelissolo A (1995) The benzodiazepine receptor: the enigma of the endogenous ligand. *Encephale* 21: 133–140

9 Jochemsen R, Breimer DD (1984) Pharmacokinetics of benzodiazepines: metabolic pathways and plasma level profiles. *Curr Med Res Opin* 8, Suppl 4: 60–79

10 Ginestet D (1983) Consumption of benzodiazepines: good and bad uses. *Encephale* 9 (4 Suppl 2): 97B–101B

11 Norman TR, Judd FK, Marriott PF, Burrows GD (1988) Physical treatment of anxiety: the benzo-diazepines. *In*: M Roth, R Noyes, GD Burrows (eds): *Handbook of anxiety*. Elsevier Science Publishers, Amsterdam, 335–385

12 Hoehn-Saric R (1998) Generalised anxiety disorder – guidelines for diagnosis and treatment. *CNS Drugs* 9: 85–98

13 Tsoi WF (1991) Insomnia: drug treatment. *Ann Acad Med Singapore* 20: 269–272

14 Greenblatt DJ, Shader RI (1987) Pharmacokinetics of antianxiety agents. *In*: HY Metzer (ed.): *Psychopharmacology: the third generation of progress*. Raven Press, New York, 1377–1386

15 Lader M, Petursson H (1983) Rational use of anxiolytic/sedative drugs. *Drugs* 25: 514–528

16 Oelschlager H (1989) Chemical and Pharmacologic aspects of benzodiazepines. *Schweiz Rundsch Med Prax* 78: 766–772

17 Greenblatt DJ, Wright CE (1993) Clinical pharmacokinetics of alprazolam. Therapeutic implications. *Clin Pharmacokinet* 224: 453–471

18 Garzone PD, Kroboth PD (1989) Pharmacokinetics of the newer benzodiazepines. *Clin Pharmacokinet* 16: 337–364

19 Greenblatt DJ, Shader RI, Abernethy DR (1983) Drug therapy. Current status of benzodiazepines. *N Engl J Med* 309: 354–358

20 Harper KW, Collier PS, Dundee JW, Scobie G, Murray T, Watkinson G, Brodie MT (1985) Age and nature of operation influence the pharmacokinetics of midazolam. *Brit J Anaesth* 57: 866–871

21 MacGilchrist AJ, Birnie GG, Cook A, Scobie G, Murray T, Watkinson G, Brodie MT (1986) Pharmacokinetics and pharmacodynamics of intravenous midazolam in patients with severe alco-holic cirrhosis. *Gut* 27: 190–195

22 Ochs HR, Greenblatt DJ, Verburg-Ochs B, Matlis R (1986) Temazepam clearance unaltered in cir-rhosis. *Amer J Gastroenterol* 81: 80–84

23 Greenblatt DJ, Harmatz JS, Shader RI (1991) Clinical pharmacokinetics of anxiolytics and hyp-notics in the elderly. Therapeutic considerations. *Clin Pharmacokinet,* 21: 165–177

24 Richelson E (1998) Pharmacokinetic interactions of antidepressants. *J Clin Psychiat* 59 Suppl 10: 22–6

25 Greenblatt DJ, von Moltke LL, Harmatz JS, Harrel LM, Tobias S, Shader RI, Wright CE (1995) Interaction of triazolam and ketoconazole. *Lancet* 345: 191

26 Greenblatt DJ, Wright CE, Von Moltke LL, Harmatz JS, Ehrenberg BL, Harrel LM, Corbett K, Counihan M, Tobias S, Shader RI (1998) Ketoconazole inhibition of triazolam and alprazolam clearance: differential kinetic and dynamic consequences. *Clin Pharmacol Ther* 64: 237–247

27 Hulhoven R, Desager JP, Cox S, Harvengt C (1988) Influence of repeated administration of cime-tidine on the pharmacokinetics and pharmacodynamics of adinazolam in healthy subjects. *Eur J Clin Pharmacol* 35: 59–64

28 Luurila H, Olkkola KT, Neuvonen PJ (1996) Interaction between erythromycin and the benzodi-azepines diazepam and flunitrazepam. *Pharmacol Toxicol* 78: 117–122

29 Yasui N (1996) The relationship between single oral dose kinetics of alprazolam and cytochrome P450 3A and cytochrome P450 2C19. *Nihon Shinkei Seishin Yakurigaku Zasshi* 16: 109–12

30 Furukori H, Otani K, Yasui N, Kondo T, Kaneko S, Shimoyama R, Ohkubo T, Nagasaki T, Sugawara K (1998) Effect of carbamazepine on the single oral dose pharmacokinetics of alprazo-lam. *Neuropsychopharmacology* 18: 364–9

31 Backman JT, Olkkola KT, Neuvonen PJ (1996) Rifampin drastically reduces plasma concentra-tions and effects of oral midazolam. *Clin Pharmacol Ther* 59: 7–13

32 Backman JT, Olkkola KT, Laasksovirta H, Neuvonen PJ (1996) Concentrations and effects of oral midazolam are greatly reduced in patients treated with carbamazepine or phenytoin. *Epilepsia* 37: 253–257

33 Dorian P, Sellers EM, Kaplan HL, Hamilton C, Greenblat DJ, Abernethy D (1985)Triazolam and ethanol interaction: kinetic and dynamic consequences. *Clin Pharmacol Ther* 37: 558–562

34 Jackson CW, Markowitz JS, Brewerton TD (1995) Delirium associated with clozapine and benzodiazepine combinations. *Ann Clin Psychiat* 7: 139–141

35 Greenblatt DJ, Preskorn SH, Cotreau MM, Horst WD, Harmatz JS (1992) Fluoxetine impairs clearance of alprazolam but not clonazepam. *Clin Pharmacol Ther* 52: 479–486

36 Sproule BA, Naranjo CA, Bremner KE, Hassan PC (1997) Selective serotonin reuptake inhibitors and CNS drug interactions – a critical review of the evidence. *Clin Pharmacokinet* 33: 454–471

37 Ketter TA, Flockhart DA, Post RM, Denicoff K, Pazzaglia PJ, Marangell LB, George MS, Callahan AM (1995) The emerging role of cytochrome P450 3A in psychopharmacology. *J Clin Pharmacol* 15: 387–398

38 Munjack DJ, Baltazar PL, Bohn PB, Cabe DD, Appleton AA (1990) Clonazepam in the treatment of social phobia: a pilot study. *J Clin Psychiat* 51 Suppl.: 35–40, discussion 50–53

39 Ontiveros A, Fontaine R (1990) Social phobia and clonazepam. *Can J Psychiat* 35: 439–441

40 Davidson JR, Ford SM, Smith RD, Potts NL (1991) Long term treatment of social phobia with clonazepam. *J Clin Psychiat* 52 Suppl.: 16–20

41 Davidson JR, Potts N, Richichi E, Krishnan R, Ford SM, Smith R, Wilson WH (1991) Treatment of social phobia with clonazepam and placebo. *J Clin Psychopharmacol* 13: 423–428

42 Bodkin JA, White K (1989) Clonazepam in the treatment of obsessive compulsive disorder associated with panic disorder in one patient. *J Clin Psychiat* 50: 265–266

43 Hewlett WA, Vinogradov S, Agras WS (1992) Clomipramine, clonazepam and clonidine treatment of obsessive compulsive disorder. *J Clin Psychopharmacol* 12: 420–430

44 Gelpin E, Bonne O, Peri T, Brandes D, Shalev AY (1996) Treatment of recent trauma survivors with benzodiazepines: a prospective study. *J Clin Psychiat* 57: 390–394

45 Tyrer P, Seivewright N, Murphy S, Ferguson B, Kingdon D, Barczak P, Brothwell J, Darling C, Gregory S, Johnson AL (1988) The Nottingham study of neurotic disorder: comparison of drug and psychological treatments. *Lancet* 2: 235–240

46 Rosenbaum JF (1982) The drug treatment of anxiety *N Engl J Med* 306: 401–4

47 Laux G (1995) Current status of treatment with benzodiazepines. *Nervenarzt* 66: 311–322

48 Busch FN, Miller FT, Weiden PJ (1989) A comparison of two adjunctive treatment strategies in acute mania. *J Clin Psychiat* 50: 453–5

49 Sachs GS, Rosenbaum JF, Jones L (1990) Adjunctive clonazepam for maintenance treatment of bipolar affective disorder. *J Clin Psychopharmacol* 10: 42–7

50 Lenox RH, Newhouse PA, Creelman WL, Whitaker TM (1992) Adjunctive treatment of manic agitation with lorazepam versus haloperidol: a double-blind study. *J Clin Psychiat* 53: 47–52

51 Kusumakar V, Yatham LN, Haslam DR, Parikh SV, Matte R, Silverstone PH, Sharma V (1997) Treatment of mania, mixed state, and rapid cycling. *Can J Psychiat* 42 Suppl 2: 79S–86S

52 Lejoyeux M, Solomon J, Ades J (1998) Benzodiazepine treatment for alcohol dependent patients. *Alcohol* 33: 563–575

53 Schaffer A, Naranjo CA (1998) Recommended drug treatment strategies for the alcoholic patient. *Drugs* 56: 571–585

54 Weissman MM, Prusoff B, Sholomskas AJ, Greenwald S (1992) A double-blind clinical trial of alprazolam, imipramine, or placebo in the depressed elderly. *J Clin Psychopharmacol* 12: 175–82

55 Casacalenda N, Boulenger JP (1998) Pharmacologic treatments effective in both generalised anxiety disorder and major depressive disorder – clinical and theoretical implications. *Can J Psychiat* 43: 722–730

56 Sussman N (1998) Anxiolytic antidepressant augmentation. *J Clin Psychiat* 59 Suppl 5: 42-8; discussion 49–50

57 Hindmarch I (1980) Psychomotor function and psychoactive drugs. *Brit J Clin Pharmacol* 10: 189–209

58 Murray JB (1984) Effects of valium and librium on human psychomotor and cognitive functions. *Genet Psychol Monogr* 109: 167–197

59 Ellinwood EH Jr, Nikaido AM, Heatherly DG, Bjornsson TD (1987) Benzodiazepine pharmacodynamics: evidence for biophase rate limiting mechanisms. *Psychopharmacology (Berl)* 91: 168–74

60 Lader M (1994) Benzodiazepines: a risk benefit profile. *CNS Drugs* 1: 377–387

61 Hinrichs JV, Mewaldt SP, Ghoneim MM, Berie JL (1982) *Pharmacol Biochem Behav* 17: 165–170

62 Taylor JL, Tinklenberg JR (1987) Cognitive impairment and benzodiazepines. *In*: HY Meltzer (ed.): *Psychopharmacology: the third generation of progress*. Raven Press, New York, 1449–1454

63 Barbee JG (1993) Memory, benzodiazepines, and anxiety: integration of theoretical and clinical perspectives. *J Clin Psychiat* 54 Suppl: 86–97; discussion 98–101

64 Roache JD, Griffiths RR (1985) Comparison of triazolam and pentobarbital: performance impairment, subjective effects and abuse liability. *J Pharmacol Exp Ther* 234: 120–33

65 Mejo SL (1992) Anterograde amnesia linked to benzodiazepines. *Nurse Pract* 17: 49–50

66 Braun P, Greenberg D, Dasberg H, Lerer B (1990) Core symptoms of post-traumatic stress disorder unimproved by alprazolam treatment. *J Clin Psychiat* 51: 236–238

67 Brown CR (1978) The use of benzodiazepines in prison populations. *J Clin Psychiat* 39: 219–22

68 Marrosu F, Marrosu G, Rachel MG, Biggio G (1987) Paradoxical reactions elicited by diazepam in children with classic autism. *Funct Neurol* 2: 355–61

69 Martinez-Telleria A, Cano ME, Carlos R (1992) Paradoxical reaction to midazolam after its use as a sedative in regional anesthesia *Rev Esp Anestesiol Reanim* 39: 379–80

70 O'Sullivan GH, Noshirvani H, Basoglu M, Marks IM, Swinson R, Kuch K, Kirby M (1994) Safety and side-effects of alprazolam. Controlled study in agoraphobia with panic disorder. *Brit J Psychiat* 165: 79–86

71 van der Bijl P, Roelofse JA (1991) Disinhibitory reactions to benzodiazepines: a review. *J Oral Maxillofac Surg* 49: 519–23

72 Petursson H (1994) The benzodiazepine withdrawal syndrome. *Addiction* 89: 1455–1459

73 Tyrer P (1993) Benzodiazepine dependence: a shadowy diagnosis. *Biochem Soc Symp* 59: 107–119

74 Kunovac JL, Stahl SM (1995) Future directions in anxiolytic pharmacotherapy. *Psychiat Clin N Amer* 18: 895–909

75 Morton S, Lader M (1992) Alpidem and lorazepam in the treatment of patients with anxiety disorders: comparison of physiological and psychological effects. *Pharmacopsychiatry* 25: 177–181

76 Lydiard RB, Ballenger JC, Rickels K (1997) A double-blind evaluation of the safety and efficacy of abecarnil, alprazolam, and placebo in outpatients with generalized anxiety disorder. Abecarnil Work Group. *J Clin Psychiat* 58 Suppl 11: 11–8

77 Aufdembrinke B (1998) Abercarnil, a new beta-carboline, in the treatment of anxiety disorders. *Brit J Psychiat* 173 (Suppl 34): 55–63

78 Busto U, Kaplan HL, Zawertalio L, Sellers EM (1994) Pharmacologic effects and abuse liability of bretazenil, diazepam and alprazolam in humans. *Clin Pharmacol Ther* 55: 451–463

Buspirone

Darius K. Shayegan[1] and Stephen M. Stahl[2]

[1] *Clinical Neuroscience Research Center, 8899 University Center Lane, Suite 130, San Diego, California 92122, USA*
[2] *Department of Psychiatry, University of California San Diego, USA*

Introduction

Originally envisioned as a novel antipsychotic agent [1], buspirone {8-[4-[4-(2-pyrimidinyl)-1-pipirazinyl]butyl]-8-azapiro[4, 5]decane-7,9-dione} failed to show antipsychotic efficacy in ten hospitalized schizophrenic inpatients receiving a mean dose of 1,470 mg [2]. On the contrary, a growing appreciation for buspirone's unexpected anxiolytic, but not antipsychotic properties [3, 4] ultimately influenced the nature of its prospective development. The clinical observations of buspirone's anxiolytic and subsequently discovered antidepressant effects have been correlated with the compound's acute agonist properties at serotonin (5HT, or 5-hydroxytryptamine) 1A receptors at serotonergic synapses in the dorsal raphe nucleus and hippocampus [5–7]. Thus, the potent 5-HT1A agonist buspirone (Buspar) made its U.S. debut in 1986 as a non-benzodiazepine anxiolytic of the azapirone class. Buspirone is the first, and as yet only member of the azapirone family to achieve an approved indication for the treatment of generalized anxiety disorder (GAD). Several other azapirones have been tested, and some continue in clinical development (e.g. gepirone and tandospirone), while others have been dropped from further development (e.g. transdermal buspirone and ipsapirone). The following is primarily a discussion of the neuropharmacologic mechanisms and relevant clinical implications of buspirone's theorized attenuation of central serotonergic neurotransmission in regard to defining therapeutic efficacy for generalized anxiety disorder (GAD), for disorders encompassing states of mixed anxiety/depression (MAD) including those with subsyndromal features and for major depressive disorder (MDD). The validity and clinical advantage of the widespread use of buspirone augmentation of antidepressants will also be reviewed.

Mechanism of action of buspirone: clinically relevant serotonergic pharmacodynamics

Very few available psychotropic agents enjoy an extensively documented, unequivocally understood mechanism of action. Buspirone is certainly no exception. Although *complete* characterization of buspirone's therapeutic mechanism of action is not at hand, a great deal of clinically relevant, neurobiologically-driven hypotheses concerning such mechanisms have guided the development of effective buspirone pharmacotherapies with a moderate degree of success. Perhaps the most relevant portrayal of buspirone's treatment efficacy lies within its serotonergic pharmacodynamics (see Levine and Potter, this volume).

Buspirone exhibits near-full agonist actions upon presynaptic 5-HT1A autoreceptors present on the dendrites and soma of serotonergic neurons present in the raphe nuclei (so-called presynaptic somatodendritic 5HT1A autoreceptors) [5, 6]. In this presynaptic environment, buspirone can be thought to act as a kind of "mock" serotonin, which indeed binds 5-HT1A somatodendritic autoreceptors with marked affinity. In terms of relating the therapeutic influence of buspirone with its actions in the central nervous system, buspirone's full-agonist "bluff" at presynaptic 5-HT1A autoreceptors seems sufficient to mimic the activity of endogenous serotonin at these sites. Thus, buspirone inhibits neuronal firing of the serotonergic neuron, just as 5HT itself does, when either binds to these receptor sites.

The 5-HT1A somatodendritic autoreceptors enable the presynaptic serotonin neuron to carry out a functional set of "checks and balances," as a means of ensuring the viability of its neuronal firing [7, 8]. Serotonin molecules that bind to presynaptic somatodendritic 5-HT1A autoreceptors are believed to provide the neuron with a message depicting the current state of synaptic neurotransmission (the "check" on neuronal status), whereupon sufficient receptor stimulation by these serotonin molecules is thought to then invoke a complementary cellular response of inhibiting further neuronal firing and serotonin release (the "balance"). Thus, 5-HT1A somatodendritic autoreceptors provide the presynaptic serotonergic neuron with the computational machinery capable of regulating its own neurotransmitter release, based upon synaptic cues.

Furthermore, the mechanism of information processing possessed by a neuron requires the availability of a reliable cellular conduit for signal transduction. In the case of serotonergic neurons in the dorsal raphe, neuronal signaling is thought to involve a trimeric G protein with which the 5-HT1A somatodendritic autoreceptor is co-associated [9–11]. G protein mediated activation or inhibition of second messenger systems, particularly cyclic AMP, lead ultimately to transduction of the extracellular serotonin signal into a variety of intracellular responses, including gene expression [12]. Thus, 5HT can potentially regulate the expression of its own 5HT1A receptors, as well as other gene products [13].

In theory, generalized anxiety disorder may be a state of excess serotonergic neurotransmission, perhaps due to a defective 5HT1A receptor "brake" or defective compensatory somatodendritic serotonin release [5, 6]. Restoration of buspirone to 5HT1A somatodendritic autoreceptors would thus afford a clinically desirable avenue for normalizing potentially hyperactive serotonergic neurotransmission in the dorsal raphe, a factor long suspected to contribute to the disease pathology of several anxiety disorders [5, 14].

On the other hand, serotonin "starved" synapses are theoretically associated with the disease pathology of depressive states, perhaps due in part to deficiencies of serotonin release due to overly sensitive somatodendritic autoreceptors [5, 15]. Bearing in mind the concept of buspirone as "mock" serotonin, one might associate the presence of such a ligand at serotonin-depleted receptors in at least two scenerios. At post-synaptic 5HT1A receptors, buspirone acts as a partial agonist, and thus may partially replete serotonergic function there [16]. Perhaps more importantly, at presynaptic somatodendritic 5HT1A autoreceptors, buspirone acts as a "fuller" (i.e. less partial) agonist [17] where it may exploit the transduction of information originating from its occupancy of these receptors in the extracellular milieu, into an intracellular message that propagates through the molecular machinery of the neuron *via* enzymatic cascade, ultimately to the level of the nucleus and neuronal DNA. Although the presynaptic 5-HT1A somatodendritic autoreceptor population acts acutely as a "brake" to inhibit neuronal firing, the long-term effect of continuous braking would lead to an adaptation to this dampening of serotonergic neurotransmission by the eventual decrease in presynaptic autoreceptor density. When such 5HT1A receptors are thus down-regulated, the neuron is no longer inhibited: rather, it is *disinhibited*, and neuronal firing is "turned on." This theoretically restores serotonin to "starved" synapses, and leads to an antidepressant action in a manner analogous to the mechanism of action of inhibitors of serotonin reuptake, such as the SSRIs (serotonin selective reuptake inhibitors) [18, 19].

Mechanism of action of buspirone: clinically relevant "non-serotonergic" pharmacology

The alpha2-adrenergic antagonist properties of one of buspirone's major metabolites, 1- pyrimidinylpiperazine (1-PP) [20, 21], may also facilitate the elevation of mood. 1-PP potentiates neurotransmission exclusively by blocking α-2 presynaptic adrenergic receptors on both serotonergic and noradrenergic nerve terminals, thus *disinhibiting* both norepinephrine and serotonin release. This is analogous to the mechanism of action of mirtazapine, a confirmed antidepressant with alpha 2 antagonist properties [22–24]. Thus, the alpha 2 antagonist properties of buspirone's 1-PP metabolite may also contribute to antidepressant actions of buspirone. It may also explain why buspirone may potentiate antidepressants when given as an augmenting agent, as alpha 2 antagonist properties would be theoretically synergistic with serotonin and norepinephrine reuptake blockade, just as mirtazapine can be synergistic with reuptake blockers for the treatment of resistant depression [25].

Therefore, although this mechanism remains speculative at present, it may not be so farfetched to consider possible antidepressant and anxiolytic effects resulting from buspirone's *indirect* enhancement of noradrenergic neuronal firing in the locus coeruleus. A recent clinical study conducted by Lechin et al.

(1998) offers the possible interpretation of buspirone's peripherally triggered increase in plasma noradrenaline, as a direct reflection its modification of central noradrenergic activity [26]. In healthy subjects, plasma neurotransmitter measurements in response to buspirone challenge, resulted in increased plasma noradrenaline concentration, with no rise in plasma adrenaline levels. Upon administration of buspirone in anxious patients, however, plasma adrenaline concentration increased, and elevation of plasma noradrenaline was not observed in comparison to normal subjects until buspirone administration was additionally prolonged. Although still quite preliminary, such studies concerning peripheral responses to buspirone offer another enlightening avenue of insight into a potential explanation of the mechanism of this azapirone's overall anxiolytic profile.

Pharmacokinetics of drug interactions for buspirone

Buspirone has excellent absorption upon oral-dose administration; however its typical bioavailability is rather low (approximately 4%), due to comprehensive first-pass metabolism in the liver [27]. As of this writing, the specific Cytochrome P450 (CYP) enzymes responsible for the metabolism of buspirone have not been identified. However, interaction of buspirone with drugs that alter the induction or availability of CYP450 enzyme 3A4 yields important empirical insight into the possible mechanisms involved in buspirone's biotransformation.

Many anti-infective agents, such as itraconazole and erythromycin, are potent inhibitors of CYP3A4, and likewise are known to cause clinically significant elevations in the plasma concentration of drugs that utilize 3A4 hepatic oxidation. In the case of buspirone, interactions with itraconazole and erythromycin effectively increase the azapirone's total AUC (area under the curve) 19-fold and 6-fold, respectively [28]. Common clinically observable consequences of robust 3A4 inhibition during a trial of buspirone administration include the enhancement or prolonging of both the therapeutic profile and adverse effects beyond what is normally expected of buspirone at any given dose. Similar plasma fluctuations resulting from interaction with verapamil and diltiazem have also been observed. Reduction in the tolerability to buspirone has also been observed when administered concomitantly with the weak 3A4 inhibitor nefazodone in antidepressant augmentation trials.

As standard logic would predict, the converse is true for agents that induce CYP450 enzyme 3A4. 3A4 inducers are indeed potent augmentors of buspirone metabolism, and may effectively sabotage both the therapeutic and adverse effects of buspirone treatment. One documented, and particularly powerful inducer of CYP450 3A4 is the antibiotic, rifampicin [29].

Buspirone as a generalized anxiolytic: buspirone *versus* the benzodiazepines

Benzodiazepines have long demonstrated a generally safe and effective anxiolytic profile. However, their particular mechanism of action has proven to cause undesirable long-term consequences of stimulating benzodiazepine receptors and increasing chloride conductance *via* allosteric modulation of GABA-A receptors, such as the relatively high potential for abuse and/or dependence, withdrawal, negative interaction with alcohol, and cognitive and psychomotor impairment [20, 30]. Such effects are not associated with anxiolytics of the azapirone class such as buspirone, due to their discrete therapeutic mechanism involving partial agonist actions at 5HT1A receptors in the dorsal raphe [31].

The specific sedative properties of benzodiazepines also appear to differ in nature compared to those manifested by buspirone. Several studies have shown the ability of patients to distinguish between the feeling of sedation induced by buspirone and benzodiazepine anxiolytics [32–35]. Patients treated with buspirone also appear to be more cognizant of their psychomotor impairment resulting from consumption of alcohol, than are subjects treated with benzodiazepines [36]. Buspirone's predominantly 5-HT1A mechanism of action spares anxious patients much of the withdrawal, cognitive "clouding", anterograde memory impairment, respiratory depression, cardiotoxic and overdose toxicity commonly associated with benzodiazepines [37].

One of the earliest clinical trials of buspirone made note of its positive anxiolytic effects in comparison to diazepam, in patients meeting DSM II (American Psychiatric Association 1968) criteria for anxiety [38]. Subsequent larger-scale studies of buspirone against placebo further document its effectiveness in mitigating symptoms of anxiety. The majority of these "large" subject population (i.e. N > 60) double-blind, randomized clinical investigations have documented buspirone's clinical efficacy as equal to that of standard benzodiazepines in the treatment of GAD. A more recent, meta-analysis of eight studies comprising 520 patients with GAD clearly illustrates buspirone's therapeutic features over placebo [39].

Smaller, short-term clinical trials of buspirone for the treatment of GAD and other less clearly specified states of chronic anxiety tend not to confirm the equal efficacy with benzodiazepines depicted from larger, long-term studies. As a consequence of their duration, short-term investigations of buspirone in chronic and persistent anxiety (GAD), may produce somewhat of a misconception in regards to providing a *meaningful* definition of clinical efficacy. Buspirone's anxiolytic efficacy may in fact increase over time. An open study of buspirone in patients with GAD reported approximately 50% improvement at around 3 months of treatment, with an increase to approximately 70% improvement over a total of 6 months treatment [40]. In terms of clinical anxiolytic efficacy in the treatment of GAD, buspirone has been demonstrated to be as effective as traditional benzodiazapine monotherapy [41].

Clinical pearls about the use of buspirone for the management of generalized anxiety

Because of withdrawal symptoms when benzodiazepines are discontinued, it can be difficult to switch patients from chronic benzodiazepine treatment to busprione. Although a consensus is indeed lacking, many clinicians prefer stabilizing the patient on both buspirone and the benzodiazepine for several weeks before beginning the benzodiazepine tapering process (Sussman, 1987]. Buspirone has no withdrawal properties, indeed it may be able to reduce symptoms of anxiety during benzodiazepine withdrawal. Chiaie et al. has reported promising success of buspirone over placebo, in mitigating withdrawal effects incurred from the discontinuation of lorazepam in subjects suffering from GAD [42].

Age-related physiological changes in most geriatric patients do not appear to disrupt, or alter significantly the pharmacokinetics of buspirone. Thus, using buspirone in the elderly does not generally require dosage adjustment. Since the elderly constitute a large percentage of the anxious patient population, and these patients may be the least well-equipped to bear the burdens of excessive sedation and impaired cognitive/psychomotor functioning that can be associated with benzodiazepine treatment, buspirone may have a special niche in the treatment of anxiety in the elderly. Furthermore, benzodiazepines but not busprione have become notoriously associated with fall-related injuries and motor-vehicle accidents in anxious elderly patients [43–45]. Buspirone also lacks the ability of benzodiazepines to depress respiratory functioning, which is certainly desirable for anxious patients with concomitant pulmonary disease.

Benzodiazepine pharmacotherapy in anxious elderly patients may also pose another danger. Sedation may decompensate comorbid conditions either when caused by the benzodiazepine itself, or when caused by drug interactions with concomitant medications. This may be particularly so for Alzheimer's dementia, schizophrenia in the elderly, and geriatric depression. Buspirone may thus be a preferred treatment for comorbid anxiety in such patients. Additionally, buspirone appears not to adversely affect Parkinson's disease, nor interact with antiparkinsonian agents [46, 47]. Also, buspirone lacks drug interactions with medications likely to be associated with treatment of numerous medical disorders in the elderly. It may thus be safest to avoid benzodiazepine anxiolytic regimens in such patients when less cognitively impairing compounds, such as buspirone, exist.

Case reports have indicated buspirone as being particularly effective in mitigating agitation in demented patients [48–50]. Initial dosing has been suggested to start at 5 mg three times daily, and may be titrated upwards to 20 mg three times a day [51]. Additionally, a net 22% reduction in agitated symptoms was reported by Sakauye et al. [52], in an open-label trial of buspirone in ten demented Alzheimer's patients with pronounced behavioral disturbances. Thus the potential of buspirone to cause significantly less cognitively compromising and motor-coordination impairing side-effects, in combination with its particular efficacy in mitigating behavioral problems associated with Alzheimer's dementia, has allowed it to become a favorable alternative to benzodiazepines for the management of anxiety in elderly patients, both inside and outside psychiatric practice.

Use of buspirone for mixed anxiety-depression (MAD) and subsyndromal MAD

Diagnostic criteria compiled in the DSM IV and ICD-10 in conjunction with approved indications for anxiolytic and antidepressant pharmacotherapies can suggest a clear demarcation between anxiety and depression. It has, however, been indicated that the majority of patients diagnosed with generalized anxiety disorder also present depressive symptoms [53]. Frequent clinical observations of coexisting anxious and depressive symptoms have ultimately led to the broadening of the GAD definition to include the recognition of mixed disease states of anxiety and depression with regard to formulating plans of effective treatment. The derivation of hybrid and subsyndromal disorders of mixed-anxiety/depression has allowed alternative avenues of treatment to be explored.

For example, a recent investigation of the antidepressant efficacy of buspirone in anxiety with concomitant symptoms of depression is a randomized, double-blind, placebo-controlled multicenter trial performed by Sramek et al. [54], which selectively compiled a relatively large and well-characterized sample of GAD patients exhibiting a quantifiable level of associated depressive symptoms. All study participants scored ≥ 18 on the HAM-A and between 12 and 17 on the HAM-D. After a 6-week trial of buspirone (titrated 15 to 45 mg/day) or placebo, buspirone-treated subjects averaged a 12.4-point reduction from their baseline total HAM-A score of 24.9, while patients treated with placebo averaged a reduction of 9.5-points from their mean baseline total HAM-A score of 25.6. The difference in HAM-A reductions between treatment groups was indeed significant ($p < .03$). Buspirone patients also decreased their HAM-D scores an average of 5.7 points from their mean baseline total HAM-D score of 15.8, while placebo subjects averaged a 3.5-point reduction from their mean baseline total HAM-D score of 16.3 ($p < .05$). These results favor the possibility of antidepressant efficacy of buspirone, especially in patients with concomitant anxiety, or mixed anxiety and depression.

Interestingly, the first of the few existing double-blind, placebo-controlled trials assessing buspirone's antidepressant properties in major depressive disorder was a study by Rickels et al. in 155 outpatients diagnosed as suffering from major depression with moderate concomitant levels of anxiety [55]. Upon finishing 8 weeks of treatment, 70% of buspirone and 35% of placebo treated patients ($p < .01$) were rated as having moderate or marked improvement. Even greater differences between buspirone and placebo ($p < .001$), were assessed in the Rickels core symptom cluster of depression. The group also reported the emergence of therapeutic actions at 4 weeks, noting that the onset of action of buspirone's antidepressant properties was relatively *slow*, in agreement with buspirone's more gradual and somewhat delayed onset of anxiolytic effects [56].

Although buspirone is not yet accepted as a first-line antidepressant monotherapy, it has proven to be more popular as an augmenting agent to antidepressants for patients with major depressive disorder who have inadequate responses to first-line antidepressants such as SSRIs.

Augmentation of antidepressants with buspirone

First off, one may ask what exactly constitutes clinically useful antidepressant augmentation? Benzodiazepine anxiolytics are most commonly recognized for their effective treatment of anxious symptoms and insomnia in depressed patients. Clinical considerations of the role for benzodiazepines in the treatment of depression support the use of these anxiolytics added to antidepressants to reduce comorbid symptoms of anxiety and insomnia, particularly early in the prescribing of an antidepressant. However, the efficacy of benzodiazepines in treating primary depressive symptomatology is not well supported [57]. Since the therapeutic contribution of benzodiazepines in the treatment of depression appears to concern largely the amelioration of bothersome symptoms but not the direct enhancement of concomitantly prescribed antidepressants to reduce core symptoms of depression such as mood, one should regard benzoodiazepine pharmacotherapy as an adjunct for managing associated symptoms, but not fundamentally as an *antidepressant* augmentation strategy. However, in the case of buspirone, it not only appears to provide a similar adjunctive role in reducing symptoms of anxiety, but also actually boosts the efficacy of first-line antidepressants in the treatment of core symptoms of depression such as mood.

Aside from its impressive track record in GAD, the effectiveness and safety associated with buspirone augmentation of pro-serotonergic antidepressants might possibly serve as its second most clinically advantageous application. In fact, the response rate of depressed patients to this combination strategy may even approach 65% [20]. Among the usual side-effects anticipated for buspirone monotherapy, namely nausea, dizziness, nervousness, and headache, the buspirone plus serotonergic antidepressant "cocktail" can cause marked excitement that can be mistaken for hypomanic/manic symptoms. Rather than an induction/exacerbation of a bipolar disorder, this may actually be a harbinger of antidepressant action. For example, the induction of hypomanic-like symptoms in elderly patients, particularly of the hyperenergized, grandiose, and euphoric variety, have been attributed to the institution of buspirone (~30 mg) as an adjunct to serotonergic antidepressant therapy in geriatric patients [58]. Similarly, Robillard and Lieff reported a similar, substantial degree of mood elevation corresponding to the addition of buspirone (15–30 mg) to either trazodone or fluvoxamine monotherapies, in three elderly patients [59]. Improvements in mood coinciding with buspirone augmentation were observed several weeks following initial adjunctive treatment in these cases, but not overt mania or unequivocal hypomania.

Perhaps the most impressive documentation of buspirone antidepressant augmentation is for co-administration with fluoxetine. However, the great majority of publications on buspirone antidepressant augmentation consist of small-scale, empirical case studies or case series, often lacking placebo-control and randomization. Nevertheless, such studies have been relatively successful in providing a moderate amount of relevant insight for useful clinical interpretation. The most common study design for both small scale and the few large-scale clinical investigations has been the addition/or replacement of buspirone pharmacotherapy in patients either who fail to respond to fluoxetine or who initially respond to fluoxetine, but experience a reduction in antidepressant efficacy over time.

Fabre, reported a "short-lived" (30–60day) restoration of antidepressant effects in a 10-patient, fluoxetine-failure population, following discontinuation of fluoxetine and subsequent institution of buspirone (40–50 mg/day) [60]. Re-introducing fluoxetine, however, while maintaining treatment with buspirone was successful in again restoring antidepressant efficacy. Of the few groups to actually mount a large-scale clinical investigation of buspirone antidepressant augmentation, Dimitriou et al., in 1996 conducted an open label study of buspirone in 30 depressed patients, all of whom were refractory to a six-weak trial of either fluoxetine, paroxetine, citalopram, or clomipramine [61, 62]. Patients were similarly treated with buspirone in combination with their formerly unsuccessful antidepressant. Following 4 months of combination therapy, approximately 46% of subjects experienced total alleviation of depressive symptoms. Thus, buspirone's augmenting actions appear to occur across the SSRI spectrum (fluoxetine, paroxetine, sertraline, fluvoxamine, and citalopram). In terms of safety, this combination appears to be generally well tolerated, although there are some reports of patients developing a very mild serotonin syndrome upon treatment with buspirone and an SSRI [63, 64].

In addition to boosting the actions of SSRIs at serotonergic synapses, it is possible that the alpha 2 antagonist properties of buspirone's metabolite 1-PP may also contribute to its augmenting efficacy, as mentioned above in the discussion of buspirone's mechanism of action. This would give a boost to both noradrenergic and serotonergic neurotransmission, analogous to the mechanism of action of the alpha 2 antagonist antidepressant mirtazapine. Interestingly, Gobert et al., has reported the enhancement of SSRI induced increases in dialysate levels of dopamine and noradrenaline, but not serotonin, by buspirone augmentation, particularly in the frontal cortex of experimental animals [65].

In addition to using buspirone to augment the antidepressant actions of serotonergic antidepressants, it may also facilitate the antiobsessional effects of

SSRIs in obsessive compulsive disorder (OCD), particularly when SSRIs are given at the higher end of their dosage ranges. Evidence supporting buspirone monotherapy for the treatment of OCD, however, is both scarce and weak [66]. Available data for buspirone as an adjunct to SSRIs for OCD also stems from case reports and small, restricted trials, many of which are contradictory to one another, predicting both efficacy [67, 68] and lack of efficacy [69]. Those OCD patients who ultimately respond to serotonergic antidepressants average only a 20 to 40% reduction in OCD symptoms, with only a small population able to achieve complete remission utilizing pharmacotherapy alone. With such a broad range of response across patients with varying severity of obsessive and compulsive symptomatology, reports of variable clinical efficacy of buspirone as an adjunct to SSRIs for OCD is not surprising. However it does seem likely that there exists a small population of patients with OCD that may benefit from combination therapy with buspirone and a pro-serotonergic antidepressant.

Closing clinical impressions

Buspirone is a novel azapirone agent with marked anxiolytic and antidepressant properties. The unique serotonergic mechanism of action of buspirone affords a clinically desirable means of "normalizing" theoretically anomalous serotonin neurotransmission. Buspirone is particularly effective in generalized anxiety disorder, is favored for treatment of chronic anxiety in those prone to substance abuse and in the elderly. Buspirone may also have efficacy in mixed states of anxiety and depression as a monotherapy, and as an augmenting agent to serotonergic antidepressants for the treatment of major depressive disorder.

Buspirone pharmacotherapy offers a clearly improved safety profile over benzodiazepines, and is free from abuse liability, and has largely replaced benzodiazepines as first-line treatment for chronic anxiety. Buspirone's low incidence of performance impairment and cognitive "clouding" are key clinical features that favor its use in active adults and especially in elderly patients. Its two to three times daily administration, and delay in onset of action are undesirable features. Some clinicians minimize buspirone's efficacy in the treatment of anxiety because of this, and buspirone is more widly prescribed in the U.S. than in many European countries. With the introduction of the first new treatment for GAD in many years, namely the antidepressant venlafaxine, it will be interesting to see the impact of this upon the treatment of GAD and its use compared to buspirone. In addition, buspirone is a popular augmenting agent to serotonergic antidepressants, particularly in the U.S. Other 5HT1A partial agonists are in clinical testing, some selective and related to the azapirone buspirone, and others of different chemical structures and accompanied by other pharmacologic actions such as serotonin 2A receptor antagonist properties. The future use of buspirone and the 5HT1A partial agonist strategy for treating anxiety, depression and resistant depression remains an area of very active clinical research.

References

1 Wu YH, Rayburn JW, Allen LE, Ferguson HC, Kissel JW (1972) Psychosedative agents. 8-(4-substituted 1-piperazinylalkyl)-8-azapiro[4,5]decane-7,9-diones. *J Med Chem* 15: 477–479

2 Sathananthan GL, Sanghvi I, Phillips N et al (1975) MJ 9022: correlation between neuroleptic potential and stereotypy. *Curr Ther Res* 18: 701–705

3 Goldberg HL, Finnerty RJ (1979) The comparative efficacy of buspirone and diazepam in the treatment of anxiety. *Amer J Psychiat* 136: 1184–7

4 Rickels K, Weisman K, Norstad N, Singer M, Stoltz D, Brown A, Danton J (1982) Buspirone and diazepam in anxiety: A controlled study. *J Clin Psychiat* 43: 81–6

5 Stahl SM (1996) *Essentail Psychopharmacology*. Cambridge University Press, Cambridge

6 Stahl SM (1997) Mixed depression and anxiety: serotonin$_{1A}$ receptors as a common pharmacological link. *J Clin Psychiat* 58 (suppl 8): 20–6

7 Levine LR, Potter WZ (2000) 5-HT1A receptors: an unkept promise? (this volume)

8 Dunlop, J; Zhang, Y; Smith, DL; Schechter, LE (1998) Characterization of 5-HT1A receptor functional coupling in cells expressing the human 5-HT1A receptor as assessed with the cytosensor microphysiometer. *J Pharmacol Toxicol Meth* 40(1): 47–55

9 Dupuis, DS; Pauwels, PJ; Radu, D; Hall, H (1999) Autoradiographic studies of 5-HT1A-receptor-stimulated [35S] GTPgammaS-binding responses in the human and monkey brain. *Eur J Neurosci* 11(5): 1809–17

10 Dupuis, DS; Palmier, C; Colpaert, FC; Pauwels, PJ (1998) Autoradiography of serotonin 5-HT1A receptor-activated G proteins in guinea pig brain sections by agonist-stimulated [35S]GTPgammaS binding. *J Neurochem* 70(3): 1258–68

11 Pauwels, PJ; Tardif, S; Wurch, T; Colpaert, FC (1997) Stimulated [35S]GTP gamma S binding by 5-HT1A receptor agonists in recombinant cell lines. Modulation of apparent efficacy by G-protein activation state. *Naunyn-Schmied Arch Pharmacol* 356(5): 551–61

12 Schoeffter, P; Bobirnac, I; Boddeke, E; Hoyer, D (1997) Inhibition of cAMP accumulation *via* recombinant human serotonin 5-HT1A receptors: considerations on receptor effector coupling across systems. *Neuropharmacology* 36(4–5): 429–37

13 Lembo, PM; Ghahremani, MH; Morris, SJ; Albert, PR (1997) A conserved threonine residue in the second intracellular loop of the 5-hydroxytryptamine 1A receptor directs signaling specificity. *Mol Pharmacol* 52(1): 164–71

14 Lucki, I (1996) Serotonin receptor specificity in anxiety disorders. *J Clin Psychiat* 57 Suppl 6: 5–10

15 Eison AS, Eison MS (1994) Serotonergic mechanisms in anxiety. *Prog Neuropsychopharmacol Biol Psychiat* 18: 47–62

16 Okazawa, H; Yamane, F; Blier, P; Diksic, M (1999) Effects of acute and chronic administration of the serotonin1A agonist buspirone on serotonin synthesis in the rat brain. *J Neurochem* 72(5): 2022–31

17 Rotondo, A; Nielsen, DA; Nakhai, B; Hulihan-Giblin, B; Bolos, A; Goldman, D (1997) Agonist-promoted down-regulation and functional desensitization in two naturally occurring variants of the human serotonin1A receptor. *Neuropsychopharmacology* 17(1): 18–26

18 Schreiber R, De Vry J (1993) 5-HT1A receptor ligands in animal models of anxiety, impulsivity, and depression: multiple mechanisms of action? *Prog Neuropsychopharmacol Biol Psychiat* 17: 87–104

19 Baldwin DS, Birtwistle J (2000) Selective serotonine re-uptake inhibitors in anxiety disorders: room for improvement. (this volume)

20 Sussman N (1998) Anxiolytic antidepressant augmentation. *J Clin Psychiat* 59 (Suppl. 5): 42–8

21 Cao, BJ; Rodgers, RJ (1997) Comparative behavioural profiles of buspirone and its metabolite 1-(2-pyrimidinyl)-piperazine (1-PP) in the murine elevated plus-maze. *Neuropharmacology* 36(8): 1089–97

22 Stimmel, GL; Dopheide, JA; Stahl, SM (1997) Mirtazapine: an antidepressant with noradrenergic and specific serotonergic effects. *Pharmacotherapy* 17(1): 10–21

23 Gorman, JM (1999) Mirtazapine: clinical overview. *J Clin Psychiat* 60 Suppl 17: 9–13; discussion 46–8

24 Stahl SM (1997) *Psychopharmacology of antidepressants*. Martin Dunitz, London

25 Carpenter, LL; Jocic, Z; Hall, JM; Rasmussen, SA; Price, LH (1999) Mirtazapine augmentation in the treatment of refractory depression. *J Clin Psychiat* 60(1): 45–9

26 Lechin F, Van Der Dijs, B, Jara H, Orozco B, Baez S, Benaim M, Lechin M, Lechin A (1998) Effects of buspirone on plasma neurotransmitters in healthy subjects. *J Neural Transm* 105: 561–73

27 Mayol RF, Adamson DS, Gammans RE, LaBuddle JA (1985) Pharmacokinetics and disposition of ^{14}C-buspirone HCL after intravenous and oral dosing in man. *Clin Pharmacol Ther* 37: 210

28 Kivistö KT, Lamberg TS, Kantola T, Neuvonen PJ (1997) Plasma buspirone concentrations are greatly increased by erythromycin and itraconazole. *Clin Pharmacol Ther* 62: 348–354

29 Kivistö KT, Lamberg TS, Neuvonen PJ (1998) Concentrations and effects of buspirone are considerably reduced by rifampicin. *Brit J Clin Pharmacol* 45: 381–385

30 Eison AS, Eison MS (1984) Buspirone: as a midbrain modulator: anxiolysis unrelated to traditional benzodiazepine mechanisms. *Drug Dev Res* 4: 109–119

31 Eison MS (1990) Azapirones: mechanism of action in anxiety and depression. *Drug Therapy Supplement* August 1990: 3–8

32 Lader M (1982) Psychological effects of buspirone. *J Clin Psychiat* 43 (Sec. 2): 62–7

33 Erwin CW, Linnoila M, Hartwell J, et al (1986) Effects of buspirone and diazepam, alone and in combination with alcohol on unskilled performance and evoked potentials. *J Clin Psychopharmacol* 6: 199–209

34 Mattila M, SeppalaT, Mattila MJ (1986) Combined effects of buspirone and diazepam on objective and subjective tests of performance in healthy volunteers. *Clin Pharmacol Ther* 40: 620–626

35 Schaffler K, Klausnitzer W (1988) Single dose study of buspirone versus diazepam in volunteers. *Arzneim-Forsch* 38: 282–287

36 Sussman N (1987) Treatment of anxiety with buspirone. *Psychiatric Ann* 17: 114–118

37 Cadieux RJ (1996) Azapirones: An alternative to benzodiazepines for anxiety. *Amer Fam Physician* 53(7): 2349–53

38 Goldberg HL, Finnerty RJ (1979) The comparative efficacy of buspirone and diazepam in the treatment of anxiety. *Amer J Psychiat* 136: 1184–87

39 Gammans RE, Stringfellow JC, Hvizdos AJ et al (1992) Use of buspirone in patients with generalized anxiety disorder and coexisting depressive symptoms: a meta-analysis of eight, randomized controlled trials. *Neuropsychobiology* 25: 193–201

40 Feighner JP (1987) Buspirone in the long-term treatment of generalized anxiety disorder. *J Clin Psychiat* 48 (No. 12 suppl): 3–6

41 Goa KL, Ward A (1986) Buspirone: A preliminary review of its pharmacological properties and therapeutic efficacy as an anxiolytic. *Drugs* 32: 114–29

42 Chiaie RD, Pancheri P, Casacchia M et al (1995) Assessment of the efficacy of buspirone in patients affected by generalized anxiety disorder, shifting to buspirone from prior treatment with lorazepam: a placebo-controlled, double-blind study. *J Clin Psychopharmacol* 15: 12–19

43 Sussman N, Chou JCY (1988) Current issues in benzodiazepine use of anxiety disorders. *Psychiatric Ann* 18: 139–145

44 Smiley A (1987) Effects of minor tranquilizers and antidepressants on psychomotor performance. *J Clin Psychiat* 48 (Suppl. 12): 22–8

45 Hemmelgarn B, Suissa S, Huuang A et al (1997) Benzodiazepine use and the risk of motor vehicle accident in the elderly. *JAMA* 278: 27–31

46 Gelenberg AJ (1994) Academic highlights-buspirone: seven year update. *J Clin Psychiat* 55: 222–9

47 Baughman OL (1994) The safety record of buspirone in generalized anxiety disorder (monograph). *J Clin Psychiat* 12: 37–45

48 Colenda CC (1988) Buspirone in the treatment of agitated demented patient [Letter]. *Lancet* 1: 1169

49 Markovitz PJ (1993) Treatment of anxiety in the elderly. *J Clin Psychiat* 54(5; suppl): 66–8

50 Sky AJ, Grossberg GT (1994) The use of psychotropic medication in the management of problem behaviors in the patient with Alzheimer's disease. *Psychiat Clin N Amer* 78: 811–22

51 Zayas EM, Grossberg GT (1996) Treating the agitated alzheimer patient. *J Clin Psychiat* 57 (suppl 7): 46–51

52 Sakauye K, Camp C, Ford P (1993) Effects of buspirone on agitation associated with dementia. *Amer J Geriatr Psychiatry* 1: 82–4

53 Rickels K, Schweizer E (1993) The treatment of generalized anxiety disorder in patients with depressive symptomatology. *J Clin Psychiat* 54 (1, Suppl): 20–3

54 Sramek JJ, Tansman M, Suri A, Hornig-Rohan M, Amsterdam JD, Stahl SM, Weisler RH, Cutler

NR (1996) Efficacy of buspirone in generalized anxiety disorder with coexisting mild depressive symptoms. *J Clin Psychiat* 57(7): 287–291

55 Rickels K, Amsterdam JD, Clary C, Puzzuoli G, Schweizer E (1991) Buspirone in major depression: A controlled study. *J Clin Psychiat* 52(1): 34–8

56 Rickels K, Schweizer E, Csanalosi I et al (1988) Long-term treatment of anxiety and risk of withdrawal: prospective comparison of clorazepate and buspirone. *Arch Gen Psychiat* 45: 444–450

57 Sussman N (1993) How to manage anxious patients who are depressed. *J Clin Psychiat* 54 (5-suppl.): 8–16

58 Lebert R, Pasquier F, Goudemand M, Petit H (1993) Euphoria with buspirone after flouoxetine treatment [Letter]. *Amer J Psychiat* 150: 167

59 Robillard M, Lieff S (1995) Augmentation of antidepressant therapy by buspirone: three geriatric case histories [Letter]. *Can J Psychiat* 40: 639–640

60 Fabre LF (1990) Combined buspirone-flouxetine in severe depression. 143rd Annual Meeting of *Am Psychiat Assoc*, New York, NY [Abs.] May 12–17, 1990: 191

61 Dimitriou EC (1996) Augmenting the effects of antidepressant medication by adding buspirone. Presented at the Tenth World Congress of Psychiatry, Madrid, Spain, August 23, 1996

62 Dimitriou EC, Dimitriou CE (1998) Buspirone augmentation of antidepressant therapy. *J Clin Psychopharmacol* 18(6): 465–9

63 Spigset O, Adielsson G (1997) Comorbid serotonin syndrome and hyponatraemia caused by citalopram-buspirone interaction. *Int Clin Psychopharmacol* 12: 61–3

64 Baetz M, Malcolm D (1995) Serotonin syndrome from fluvoxamine and buspirone. *Can J Psychiat* 40(7): 428–9

65 Gobert A, Rivet JM, Cistarelli JM et al (1997) Buspirone enhances duloxetine- and fluoxetine-induced increases in dialysate levels of dopamine and noradrenaline, but not serotonin, in the frontal cortex of freely moving rats. *J Neurochem* 68: 1326–29

66 Pato MT, Pigott TA, Hill JL, Grover GN, Bernstein S, Murphy DL (1991) Controlled comparison of buspirone and clomipramine in obsessive-compulsive disorder. *Amer J Psychiat* 148: 127–9

67 Jenike MA, Baer L, Buttolph L (1991) Buspirone augmentation of fluoxetine in patients with obsessive compulsive disorder. *J Clin Psychiat* 52: 13–4

68 Markowitz PJ, Stagno SJ, Calabrese JR (1990) Buspirone augmentation of fluoxetine in obsessive-compulsive disorder. *Amer J Psychiat* 147: 798–800

69 Grady TA, Pigott TA, L'Heureux F, Hill JL, Bernstein SE, Murphy DL (1993) Double-blind study of adjuvant buspirone hydrochloride for flouxetine-treated patients with obsessive compulsive disorder. *Amer J Psychiat* 150: 819–21

Anxiolytics
ed. by M. Briley and D. Nutt
© 2000 Birkhäuser Verlag/Switzerland

Tricyclic antidepressants

Rudolf Hoehn-Saric

115 Meyer Building, Johns Hopkins Hospital, Baltimore, MD 21287-7115, USA

In the middle 1950s, when imipramine, the first tricyclic antidepressant (TCA), became available, investigators did not consider that this compound might be useful in the treatment of anxiety disorders. Meprobamate and the first benzodiazepines were effective in alleviating anxiety, while imipramine given in a single dose often accentuated tension and agitation. During the later part of that decade Klein and Fink [1] observed that inpatients with "episodic anxiety," characterized by "the sudden onset of inexplicable panic attacks, accompanied by rapid breathing, palpitations, weakness, and a feeling of impending death" improved on imipramine while other sedatives and phenothiazines were ineffective. This observations led to controlled studies and to the separation of anxiety neurosis into panic disorder and generalized anxiety disorder. Imipramine was found effective in the prevention of panic attacks but not of anticipatory anxiety [2]. Subsequently, several TCAs were developed of which amitriptyline and doxepine had sedative effects. Sedative TCAs became useful in the treatment of anxious and agitated patients with depression, however, the long-term reduction of anxiety was attributed to improvement of depression, rather than to specific anxiolytic effects of TCAs. The effectiveness of imipramine and other TCAs in treatment of panic disorder led to studies of other conditions that have episodic attacks of anxiety, such as simple phobias, social phobia, post-traumatic stress disorder, and obsessive compulsive disorder. TCAs were not regarded to be useful in generalized anxiety disorder until, in the 1980s, several studies demonstrated that this disorder responded to prolonged treatment with imipramine. TCAs vary considerably in their pharmacodynamic profiles. Moreover, the effectiveness of TCAs differs in anxiety disorders. However, with appropriate choice, most chronic anxiety disorders are treatable with TCAs. The main drawback of TCAs is unpleasant and sometimes limiting side-effects. Therefore, newer antidepressants that are not necessarily more effective but have more favorable side-effect profiles, have begun to overshadow TCAs.

Pharmacological properties and mechanisms of TCAs

Pharmacodynamics of TCAs

TCAs have multiple mechanisms of action that occur over a relatively narrow concentration range. The tertiary TCAs, clomipramine, doxepine, amitriptyline and imipramine, are serotonin and norepinephrine reuptake inhibitors. The secondary TCAs, nortriptyline, desipramine and protriptyline are predominantly norepinephrine reuptake inhibitors. Tertiary TCAs are metabolized into secondary TCAs. Therefore, patients taking tertiary TCAs receive compounds that are serotonin and norepinephrine reuptake inhibitors while patients taking secondary TCAs receive compounds that are primarily norepinephrine reuptake inhibitors. In addition, TCAs are to different degrees histamine-1-receptor and muscarinic receptor antagonist, block the alpha-1-noradrenergic receptor and have quinidine-like actions on the myocardium and cardiac conduction system [3]. Tables 1 and 2 present pharmacodynamic properties of some commonly used TCAs. TCAs differ considerably in their ability to inhibit norepinephrine and serotonin reuptake or block histamine, muscarinic or alpha-adrenergic receptors. These differences modify their effectiveness in anxiety reduction and their side-effect profiles. Clomipramine is a tertiary TCA with strong serotonin reuptake inhibition and marked effects on other receptors.

Antidepressant and anti-anxiety effects of TCAs are attributed to their norepinephrine and serotonin reuptake inhibitory properties [4]. All TCAs are effective in reducing panic attack while antidepressants that are not primarily norepinephrine or serotonin reuptake inhibitors, for instance buproprion [5], are ineffective. The neuropathology of panic attacks is not fully understood and may involve the limbic system as well as several nuclei of the brain stem [6]. Among these nuclei, the noradrenergic locus coeruleus has extensive connections to other brain structures; it controls attention and maximizes relevant

Table 1. Potency of TCAs in inhibiting NE and 5HT reuptake[*]

DRUG	NE	5HT
Tertiary amines		
Doxepine	5.3	0.36
Amitriptyline	4.2	1.5
Imipramine	7.7	2.4
Secondary amines		
Nortriptyline	25	0.38
Protriptyline	100	0.36
Desipramine	110	0.29

[*] $10^{-7} \times 1/Ki$, in which Ki = inhibitory constant in molarity. The higher the number, the greater the reuptake inhibition. Modified from Richelson [3].
NE = Norepinephrine 5-HT = Serotonin

Table 2. Potency of TCAs to block some neuroreceptors[*]

DRUG	H1	Muscarinic	α-1-Adrenergic
Tertiary amines			
Doxepine	420	1.2	4.2
Amitriptyline	91	5.5	3.7
Imipramine	9.1	1.1	1.1
Secondary amines			
Nortriptyline	10	0.67	1.7
Protriptyline	4.0	4.0	0.77
Desipramine	0.91	0.5	0.77

[*] $10^{-7} \times 1/Kd$, where Kd = equilibrium dissociation constant in molarity. High affinity corresponds to high receptor blockade. Modified from Richelson [3].
H1 = Histamine-1-receptor

responses to internal and external stimuli [7]. Stimulation of the locus coeruleus leads to panic-like responses in animals and man [8]. The TCA-induced increase of norepinephrine at the alpha-2-adrenoreceptors of the locus coeruleus stabilizes its activity and decreases excessive responses. Patients receiving TCAs or the alpha-2-agonist, clonidine, may continue to experience steady tension but are relieved of excessive arousal, including panic attacks [9].

The effect of the serotonergic system on anxiety is complex. At least 17 serotonergic receptors that differ in their functions have been identified [10]. Tertiary TCAs have serotonin reuptake inhibitory qualities that increase serotonin in all serotonergic synapses. Panic attacks probably are reduced by the restraining effect of serotonin on the locus coeruleus [4]. In addition, tertiary TCAs reduce psychic symptoms of anxiety including obsessions and compulsions. These effects can be attributed to the serotonergic system, since they are most prominent in clomipramine, the TCA with strongest serotonin reuptake inhibition. We [11] found that in patients with generalized anxiety disorder, a disorder with strong psychic component, imipramine plasma levels correlated positively with anxiety reduction while desipramine plasma levels correlated negatively with improvement. Mavissakalian and Perel [12] found in patients with panic disorder positive correlations between imipramine, but not desipramine, level and the improvement of agoraphobia, a disorder with predominantly psychic symptoms. In imaging studies, medications with serotonin reuptake inhibition reduce frontal cerebral blood flow in obsessive-compulsive patients [13] and may cause apathy and indifference [14]. These findings suggest that an increase of serotonin in the brain reduces frontal lobe function, leading to reduction of fears, worries and obsessions.

Antihistaminic effects of TCAs cause sedation [15] while the blockade of the alpha 1 noradrenergic receptor causes orthostatic hypotension.

Anticholinergic effects due to blockade of muscarinic receptors cause dry mouth, constipation, difficulties urinating, increased heart rate, increased intraocular pressure, difficulties in visual accommodation and cognitive disturbances [15]. However, in patients with irritable bowel syndrome, amitriptyline produces more feelings of well being and reduces abdominal pain and satisfaction with bowel movements [16].

Quinidine-like action on the myocardium and cardiac conduction system may cause prolongation of the P-R interval, QRS complex, and the Q-T interval. In addition, ST-segment and T-wave inversion or flattening, atrial fibrillations, ventricular premature contractions, and ventricular tachycardia have been observed [17].

Pharmacokinetics of TCAs

TCAs are relatively homogenous with regard to their pharmacokinetics. They are absorbed rapidly with a maximum plasma concentration in 1 to 3 h after ingestion for tertiary amine TCAs and 4 to 8 h for secondary amine TCAs. Their half-lives in healthy individuals are 24 h or more when active metabolites are considered, with exception of protryptiline which has a longer half-life. With regular administration steady-state develops within 5 to 7 days. However, there is as much as a 30-fold interindividual variability in the rate of biotransformation and clearance of TCAs. Approximately, 7% of caucasians are slow metabolizers of TCAs because of deficiency in the hepatic enzyme 2D6. Patients over 60 years develop approximately twice the plasma TCA concentration on the same dose as younger individuals [15]. Thus, the same dose of a TCA can cause adequate, therapeutically insufficient or toxic plasma levels. Plasma levels should be obtained after steady-state has been reached, particularly when the dose appear to be therapeutically insufficient or causes disturbing side-effects. TCAs can be given in a single daily dose, usually at bedtime. In patients with poor tolerance the distribution of the dose may reduce the intensity of side-effects.

Side-effects of TCAs

The most common cardiovascular complication is orthostatic hypotension, other cardiac problem occur in less than 5% of treated patients. Tachycardia due to reduced vagal cardiac tone [18] occurs regularly and can reach 120 beats per minute. Mild increase of blood pressure is common but can reach pathological values in predisposed patients. Patients with preexisting bundle branch block are at risk to develop a heart block. On the other hand, the quinidine-like action of TCAs can improve cardiac arrhythmias [17]. Sudden death in children on TCAs has been reported but the connection between death and medication was not clearly established [19]. Fortunately, the more severe complications of TCA treatment are rare and the drugs are generally well tolerated by children and adults, even when they have cardiovascular diseases. Since cardiac symptoms correlate with plasma drug levels measuring of drug levels is recommended, particularly in the elderly. In children and patients with potential cardiac diseases one needs to obtain an electrocardiogram and, if necessary, a consultation with an internist before staring treatment.

Other complications are sexual disturbances, although clomipramine can be useful in the treatment of premature ejaculation [20]. Weight gain can become a problem and excessive sweating may be embarrassing. TCAs lower the seizure threshold and can evoke seizures in patient with negative history of epilepsy. Patients with history of seizures should receive antiepileptic medication before being placed on TCAs.

Sedation and anticholinergic effects of TCA can cause diminished attention and memory and psychomotor impairment [21]. Sedation caused by blockade of the histamine-1-receptor, but sedation decreases within 2 weeks. Higher doses, particularly in the elderly, can cause disturbing memory impairment and delirium due to the anticholinergic effects of TCAs.

In a naturalistic follow-up of panic disorder patients 35% of those patients were unable to tolerate tricyclic antidepressants and discontinued them. Early discontinuations were most commonly from overstimulation, orthostatic reactions, and allergic reactions. Late discontinuations were most common for weight gain and persistent anticholinergic reactions. Forty percent of long-term patients reported weight gain, with the mean weight gain being 22 pounds [22].

Many anxiety disorders are chronic and need long-term treatment. Even when well tolerated, TCAs caused tachycardia; elevation of blood pressure [23] and weight gain may, in the long term, unfavorably affect the health of the patient.

Sudden withdrawal of TCA may cause transitory withdrawal reactions due to rebound from their anticholinergic and serotonergic actions. Withdrawal reactions consist of nausea, lethargy, and insomnia, tremor, headache, problems with balance, anxiety, agitation and crying spells [24, 25]. They are generally milder than those seen after discontinuation of selective serotonin reuptake inhibitors and occur in a minority of patients. A gradual taper of the medication prevents withdrawal reactions.

Clinical use of TCAs

Panic disorder

Panic disorder is characterized by paroxysmal attacks of severe anxiety and prominent respiratory and cardiovascular symptoms. Attacks may occur spontaneously but are soon linked to situations in which they have occurred previously, inducing anticipatory anxiety. Avoidance of panic-inducing situations leads to agoraphobia. Fifteen controlled studies have shown that imipramine is effective in reducing panic attacks with gradual reduction of avoidance and anticipatory anxiety [26]. Substantial reduction of panic attacks occur after 4 weeks of treatment but the effects of the medication are not fully experienced until 8 to 12 weeks of treatment. Anticipatory anxiety usually diminishes after the panic attacks have been reduced. Phobic avoidance is the last to be affected and may need behavioral treatment. Other TCAs also reduce panic attacks. Clomipramine was found equal or superior to other TCAs and may be effective at slightly lower doses [28]. Studies with desipramine and nortriptyline were promising [27]. Thus, TCAs with combined serotonin and norepinephrine reuptake inhibition as well as TCAs with predominately norepinephrine reuptake inhibition prevent panic attacks when they are taken regularly.

During the first weeks of treatment, TCAs may cause tension, insomnia, anxiety, and agitation. This effect is stronger in non-sedating TCAs and is dose dependent. Anxiety disorder patients are very sensitive to side-effects of medications and tend to stop taking them when they cause discomfort. Therefore, patients should be started with a low dose, which is then increased according to individual tolerance. During the first few weeks of treatment, before TCAs suppress panic attacks and while patients feel overstimulated by the medication, constant reassurance and encouragement is necessary. Additional treatment with benzodiazepines may ease the discomfort during the initial phase of treatment. Once a panic disorder is under control visits can be reduced to brief medication checks. After treatment with imipramine 45% to 70% of patients were found to be panic free [26]. Patients with severe avoidance or with personality problems may need additional behavior or psychotherapy.

Some patients respond to smaller doses of TCAs than are effective in depression [2]. However, studies by Mavissakalian and Perel [12] showed that moderate doses of imipramine are optimal; lower levels are not better than placebo and higher levels yield no additional benefit. On dose of 2.25 mg/kg/day, 50% improvement was reached in 4 weeks and improvement continued beyond week 8 of treatment, The average dose in his study was imipramine 165 mg per day but some patients needed 300 mg per day to be free of panic attacks. Imipramine treatment, even without cognitive therapy, reduced measures of "anxiety sensitivity", showing that cognitive therapy is not necessary to "normalize" catastrophic misinterpretations of body sensations [29]. Fear, unreality and respiratory symptoms displayed the highest degree of early differentiation between effective and ineffective doses of imipramine, whereas palpitations, tingling and sweating had the most pronounced effect between weeks 4 and 6 of treatment [30].

In panic disorder, the prevention of panic attacks and the improvement of agoraphobia may not follow the same mechanisms. While panic attacks are inhibited by TCAs with norepinephrine and serotonin reuptake inhibition, agoraphobia, which consists predominantly of psychic symptoms, seems to respond better to the serotonergic than to the noradrenergic component of imipramine [12].

Since TCAs need several weeks to be fully effective medication should be tried at least for 6 to 8 weeks until judged to be ineffective and the patient changed to a different medication. The drawback of treatment with TCAs is the high dropout rate due to side-effects [22, 28].

Panic disorder is a chronic disorder. The optimal length of treatment is unknown but, in most practices, treatment is continued for a year, after which the dose is gradually reduced. Some patients remain free of panic attack or have such mild attacks that they need no further treatment with TCAs. However, a tendency for relapse remains. Such patients may have to stay on medication indefinitely.

Generalized anxiety disorder

Generalized anxiety disorder is characterized by persistent anxiety that may fluctuate in severity and becomes exaggerated by external stressors The prominent symptom of generalized anxiety disorder is excessive worry. Physical symptoms, while present, are milder than in panic disorder or center around worry about a particular organ system. Thus, psychic symptoms predominate the clinical picture in most but not all patients [31]. Non-sedating TCAs have little immediate effect on anxiety and benzodiazepines are more calming and have less side-effects than sedating TCAs. Therefore, it was thought that TCAs are not suitable for treatment of generalized anxiety. In the 1980s, Kahn et al. [32] found that in patients with anxiety neurosis, the benzodiazepine chlordiazepoxide became superior to imipramine during the first 2 weeks of treatment, but after the second week, imipramine begun to exceed the effect of chlordiazepoxide. During the same time, we compared the effects of imipramine with the benzodiazepine alprazolam in generalized anxiety disorder patients [33]. We hypothesized that generalized anxiety disorder patients who experienced strong autonomic, particularly cardiac and respiratory symptoms are phenomenologically close to panic disorder and, therefore, would respond to imipramine, while patients with predominantly psychic symptoms, namely worries, would do better on a benzodiazepine. Our results disproved our original assumption: imipramine was more effective in reducing psychic symptoms, such as excessive worrying, while alprazolam was more effective in reducing physical symptoms. This finding has been replicated by others [34]. Moreover, in several placebo-controlled studies imipramine appeared as effective or better than a benzodiazepine [32, 35].

The anxiolytic effects of imipramine manifest themselves gradually and increase over time while the effects of benzodiazepines are immediate but do not increase during subsequent weeks. Interestingly, imipramine also improved somatic symptoms while worsening blood pressure, heart rate and muscle tension [23]. It seems that imipramine induces feeling of well being which alter the perception of bodily functions. In one study in which depression was reason for exclusion, even mild, subsyndromal depressive symptoms predicted an unfavorable response to diazepam and a much more favorable response to antidepressant [36]. Sedating TCAs have stronger and more immediate anxiolytic effects but also have more undesirable anticholinergic side-effects.

TCAs have not been systematically explored in generalized anxiety disorder. Therefore, we do not know to what degree the serotonergic and to what degree the noradrenergic properties of TCAs contribute to the reduction of anxiety. In a recent study, we [11] examined the contribution of imipramine and its principal metabolite, desipramine, to anxiety reduction in generalized anxiety disorder patients. Plasma levels of imipramine, a TCA with serotonin and norepinephrine reuptake properties, correlated with improvement while plasma levels of desipramine, a TCA with predominantly noradrenergic properties, counteracted anxiety reduction. It appears that serotonin reuptake inhibition reduces psychic symptoms of anxiety while norepinephrine reuptake inhibition worsens them. This contrasts with the antipanic effects of imipramine and desipramine, which appear to be comparable. It appears that different anxiety disorders have mechanisms which respond differentially to pharmacological interventions.

The dose of TCAs in the treatment of generalized anxiety disorder can be lower than doses used in the treatment of depression or panic disorder [33]. The duration of treatment varies. Many generalized anxiety disorder patients see a physician while under stress. They often improve within a few weeks or months, after which they do not need regular medications. A subgroup of patients need long-term treatment. TCAs are useful when severe and lasting psychic symptoms are present [37]. Anticholinergic effects, which usually are undesirable, are helpful when anxiety symptoms aggravate an irritable bowel syndrome [16]. The disadvantages of TCAs are the necessity to be taking regularly, the slow onset of anxiolytic action, and side-effects. Therefore, GAD patients with milder symptoms prefer medications that act immediately and can be taken whenever needed.

Specific and social phobia

Specific phobias are characterized by an unreasonable fear of certain objects or situations that are known to be harmless The fear response can take panic-like proportions. However, studies with imipramine found the drug not to be more effective than placebo when pharmacotherapy was combined with behavior therapy [38]. Facing the feared situations remains the treatment of choice and additional treatment with TCAs is not indicated.

Social phobias are characterized by fears of situations in which the person feels to be under scrutiny. There are two types of social phobias: circumscribed and generalized social phobias [39]. Circumscribed social phobias, for instance fear of speaking or performing in public, resembles specific phobias. TCAs have not been used in the treatment of such phobias. Generalized social phobia is characterized by fear of any situation in which a person feels to be observed or scrutinized. In such patients anxiety is generalized but peaks dramatically during social encounters. Generalized social phobias are often treatment resistant. While individual case reports found TCAs useful no controlled studies with TCAs have been done. Positive results have been claimed for a large open trial with clomipramine [26], but an open trial by Simpson et al. [40] found imipramine disappointing.

Post-traumatic stress disorder

Post-traumatic stress disorder is characterized by anxiety and distress that is caused by intrusive thoughts and dreams about past traumatic events. It leads to avoidance of stimuli associated with the trauma. Persistent symptoms of increased arousal may be presented. Patients often react panic-like to trauma related stimuli and comorbid depression frequently is present. Therefore, TCAs are prescribed to patents in whom the condition has become chronic. Chronic post-traumatic stress disorder is difficult to treat and often unresponsive to interventions. The placebo response in controlled studies has been approximately 20% which is, except in obsessive-compulsive disorder, lower than in other anxiety disorders [41]. Imipramine and amitriptyline have proven to be superior to placebo in reducing intrusive thoughts, avoidance, and hyperarousal, however, the improvement is only modest [42]. With medications, most patients continue to experience symptoms but to a lesser degree. Some patients need lifelong pharmacotherapy and for them attempts to reduce the dose may lead to relapse even 20 or more years after exposure to trauma [41].

Obsessive-compulsive disorder

Intrusive thoughts, impulses or images, and repetitive behavior that a person feels driven to perform characterize obsessive-compulsive disorder. Obsessions and attempts to control compulsions cause marked anxiety or distress. DSM-IV [43] classified obsessive-compulsive disorder as an anxiety disorder although many investigators believe it to be a disorder *sui generis* [44]. The positive response to serotonin but not to norepinephrine reuptake inhibitors or to other anxiolytic supports the latter view [45]. Obsessive-compulsive disorder worsens when patients are depressed and TCAs have been used in such patients with modest efficacy. We demonstrated that in obsessive-compulsive patients who were comorbid with major depression, the predominantly norepinephrine reuptake inhibitor desipramine also reduced obsessive-compulsive symptoms, but to a lesser degree then the selective serotonin reuptake inhibitor sertraline [46]. However, studies in non-depressed patients have shown that TCAs, with exception of clomipramine, are ineffective [45]. The primary pharmacological action of clomipramine is inhibition of the serotonin reuptake pump, whereas other TCAs are relatively nonselective. However, desmethylclomipramine, the principal metabolite of clomipramine, is a norepinephrine reuptake inhibitor. In addition, clomipramine has strong antihistaminic, anticholinergic effects and blocks dopaminergic and adrenergic receptors, causing considerable degree of side-effects, which limits its use. Clomipramine has a narrow therapeutic range and doses four times higher than the recommended maximal dose can result in cardiac toxicity, seizures and even death.

Several studies have shown clomipramine to be equally effective to selective serotonin reuptake inhibitors (SSRIs) and a meta-analysis of controlled studies found clomipramine superior to SSRIs [47]. However, clomipramine was the first drug that was systematically studied in obsessive-compulsive patients. When subsequent antidepressants were studied the patient population had changed and many patients who had failed clomipramine entered those studies. Since some patients respond better to clomipramine than to SSRIs, it was thought that clomipramine's additional norepinephrine reuptake inhibitory action may yield better results than the inhibition of serotonin reuptake alone. However, the addition of desipramine to serotonin reuptake inhibitors failed to improve the outcome in one study [48]. In clinical practice, some patients respond better to clomipramine while others do better on an SSRI.

As with other TCAs, the dose of clomipramine has to be gradually increased. Most studies suggest a daily dose of 150 mg to 250 mg; higher doses, while sometimes therapeutically more effective, are not recommended because they lower the seizure threshold. At least 6 weeks of treatment are necessary to obtain significant improvement and patients continue to improve over subsequent months. In treatment-resistant patients, intravenous clomipramine, given in 14 infusions, starting with 25 mg a day and gradually increasing to 250 mg a day, led to improvement of 6 out of 25 previously inadequate responders to clomipramine [49]. Since obsessive-compulsive disorder is a chronic disorder, most seriously ill patients need to stay on medications indefinitely. Medication usually improves the symptoms and provides relief, but the majority of patients continue to experience some obsessions and compulsions.

TCAs in children and adolescents

There are few double-blind, placebo-controlled TCA studies in children and adolescents and few of them report positive results. In one study, imipramine was found to be significantly superior to placebo in the treatment of separation anxiety in children [50] but this finding was not replicated in subsequent studies with imipramine [51] and clomipramine [52]. However, clomipramine was found useful in the treatment of obsessive-compulsive children [53]. As in adults, TCAs reduce heart variability, lower vagal tone [54] and long-term uses can induce some electrocardiograph changes. Sudden unexplained death occurred in children who were stable on TCA medications, but a clear association of sudden death with TCA remains unproved. It is advisable to monitor the electrocardiogram of children on TCAs.

Conclusions

TCAs are effective in the treatment of most but not all anxiety disorders. They are most effective in panic and generalized anxiety disorder, less effective in post-traumatic stress disorder and of questionable value in phobias. Norepinephrine as well as serotonin reuptake inhibitory TCAs block panics attacks; psychic symptoms respond better to TCAs with serotonin reuptake inhibition. TCAs that are sedating have an immediate anxiolytic effect, however, the decrease of psychic symptom and of panic attacks occurs gradually over several weeks.

The advantage of TCAs is their low cost and their effectiveness in the treatment of panic disorder and generalized anxiety disorder. Patients with migraine headache or irritable bowel syndrome tolerate TCAs better than selective serotonin reuptake inhibitors. Their disadvantage is side-effects that usually are only uncomfortable but can reach dangerous proportions in predisposed individuals, particularly in the elderly. Therefore, newer antidepressants with more favorable side-effect profiles are gradually replacing TCAs. TCAs still have a solid place in the treatment of younger patient, in patients who respond poorly to other antidepressants, and in patients who cannot afford expensive new antidepressants.

References

1 Klein DF, Fink M (1962) Psychiatric reaction patterns to imipramine. *Amer J Psychiat* 119: 432–438
2 Klein DF (1981) Anxiety reconceptualized *In*: DF Klein, JG Rabkin (eds): *Anxiety: new research and changing concepts.* Raven Press, New York, 235–263
3 Richelson E (1990) Antidepressants and brain neurochemistry. *Mayo ClinProc* 65: 1227–1236
4 Frazer A (1997) Pharmacology of antidepressants. *J Clin Psychopharmacol* 17 Suppl 1: 2S–18S
5 Sheehan DV, Raj AB, Sheehan H, Soto S (1990) Is buspirone effective for panic disorder? *J Clin Psychopharmacol* 10: 1:3–11
6 Gorman JM, Liebowitz MR, Fyer AJ, Stein J (1989) A neuroanatomical hypothesis for panic disorder. *Amer J Psychiat* 146: 2:148–161
7 Aston-Jones G, Valentino RJ, Van Bockstaele EJ, Meyerson AT (1994) Locus coeruleus, stress, and PTSD: Neurobiological and clinical parallels. *In*: MM Murburg (ed.): *Catecholamine function in posttraumatic stress disorder.* American Psychiatric Press, Washington D.C., 17–62
8 Redmond DE, Huang YH (1979) II. New evidence for a locus coeruleus-norepinephrine connection with anxiety. *Life Sci* 25: 2149–2162
9 Hoehn-Saric R, Merchant AF, Keyser ML, Smith VK (1981) Effects of clonidine on anxiety disorders. *Arch Gen Psychiat* 38: 1278–1282
10 Kroeze WK, Roth BL (1998) The molecular biology of serotonin receptors: Therapeutic implications for the interface of mood and psychosis. *Biol Psychiat* 44: 1128–1142
11 McLeod DR, Hoehn-Saric R, Porges SW, Kowalski PA, Clark CM (2000) Therapeutic effects of imipramine are contraacted by its metabolite, desipramine. *J Clin Psychopharmacol; in press*

12 Mavissakalian MR, Perel JM (1989) Imipramine dose-response relationship in panic disorder with agoraphobia: Preliminary findings. *Arch Gen Psychiat* 46: 127–131

13 Hoehn-Saric R, Benkelfat C (1994) Structural and functional brain imaging in obsessive compulsive disorder. *In*: E Hollander, J Zohar, D Marazziti, B Oliver (eds): *Current insights in obsessive compulsive disorder*. John Wiley and Sons, New York, 183–211

14 Hoehn-Saric R, Lipsey JR, McLeod DR (1990) Apathy and indifference in patients on fluvoxamine and fluoxetine. *J Clin Psychopharmacol* 10: 343–345

15 Preskorn SH (1993) Pharmacokinetics of antidepressants: Why and how they are relevant to treatment. *J Clin Psychiat* 54, Suppl. 9: 14–34

16 Rajagopalan M, Kurian G, John E (1998) Symptom relief with amitiptyline in the irritable bowel syndrome. *J Gastroenterol Hepatol* 13: 738–741

17 Glassman AH, Bigger JT (1981) Cardiovascular effects of therapeutic doses of tricyclic antidepressants. *Arch Gen Psychiat* 38: 815–820

18 McLeod DR, Hoehn-Saric R, Porges SW, Zimmerli WD (1992) Effects of alprazolam and imipramine on parasympathetic cardiac control in patients with generalized anxiety disorder. *Psychopharmacology* 107: 535–540

19 Hawkridge SM, Stein DJ (1998) A risk-benefit assessment of pharmacotherapy for anxiety disorders in children and adolescents. *Drug Safety* 19: 283–297

20 Kim SC, Seo KK (1998) Efficacy and safety of fluoxetine, sertraline and clomipramine in patients with premature ejaculation: A double-blind, placebo controlled study. *J Urol* 159: 425–427

21 Deptula D, Pomara N (1990) Effects of antidepressants on human performance: A review. *J Clin Psychopharmacol* 10: 2:105–111

22 Noyes R, Garvey MJ, Cook BL (1989) Follow-up study of patients with panic disorder and agoraphobia with panic attacks treated with tricyclic antidepressants. *J Affect Disord* 16: 249–256

23 McLeod DR, Hoehn-Saric R, Zimmerli WD, De Souza E, Oliver LK (1990) Treatment effects of alprazolam and imipramine: Physiological versus subjective changes in patients with generalized anxiety disorder. *Biol Psychiat* 28: 849–861

24 Dilsaver SC (1989) Antidepressant withdrawal syndromes: Phenomenology and pathophysiology. *Acta Psychiat Scand* 79: 113–117

25 Lejoyeux M, Ades J (1997) Antidepressant discontinuation: A review of the literature. *J Clin Psychiat* 58 Suppl 7: 11–16

26 American Psychiatric Association (1998) Practice guideline for the treatment of patients with panic disorder. *Amer J Psychiat* 155, May Suppl.: 1–34

27 Jefferson JW (1997) Antidepressants in panic disorder. *J Clin Psychiat* 58 Suppl 2: 20–24

28 Papp LA, Schneier FR, Fyer AJ, Liebowitz MR, Gorman JM, Coplan JD, Campeas R, Fallon BA, Klein DF (1997) Clomipramine treatment of panic disorder: Pros and cons. *J Clin Psychiat* 58: 423–425

29 Mavissakalian M, Perel JM, Talbott-Green M, Sloan C (1998) Gauging the effectiveness of extended imipramine treatment for panic disorder with agoraphobia. *Biol Psychiat* 43: 848–854

30 Mavissakalian M (1996) Phenomenology of panic attacks: Responsiveness of individual symptoms to imipramine. *J Clin Psychopharmacol* 16: 233–237

31 Hoehn-Saric R (1998) Generalised anxiety disorder: Guidelines for diagnosis and treatment. *CNS Drugs* 9: 85–98

32 Kahn RJ, McNair DM, Lipman RS, Covi L, Rickels K, Downing R, Fisher S, Frankenthaler LM (1986) Imipramine and chlordiazepoxide in depressive and anxiety disorders II. Efficacy in anxious outpatients. *Arch Gen Psychiat* 43: 79–85

33 Hoehn-Saric R, McLeod DR, Zimmerli WD (1988) Differential effects of alprazolam and imipramine in generalized anxiety disorder: Somatic versus psychic symptoms. *J Clin Psychiat* 49: 8:293–301

34 Rocca P, Fonzo V, Scotta M, Zanalda E, Ravizza L (1997) Paroxetine efficacy in the treatment of generalized anxiety disorder. *Acta Psychiat Scand* 95: 444–450

35 Rickels K, Schweizer E (1993) The treatment of generalized anxiety disorder in patients with depressive symptomatology. *J Clin Psychiat* 54:(Suppl.): 20–23

36 Schweizer E, Rickels K (1997) Strategies for treatment of generalized anxiety in the primary care setting. *J Clin Psychiat* 58, Suppl 3: 27–31

37 Rickels K, Schweizer E (1990) The clinical course and long-term management of generalized anxiety disorder. *J Clin Psychopharmacol* 10: 3:101–109

38 Zitrin CM, Klein DF, Woerner MG (1983) Treatment of phobias, I: Comparison of imipramine and

placebo. *Arch Gen Psychiat* 40: 125–138

39 Ballenger JC, Davidson JRT, Lecrubier Y, Nutt DJ, Bobes J, Beidel DC, Ono Y, Westenberg GM (1998) Consensus statement on social anxiety disorder from the International Consensus Group on Depression and Anxiety. *J Clin Psychiat* 59 Suppl 17: 54–60

40 Simpson HB, Schneier FR, Campeas RB, Marshall RD, Fallon BA, Davies S, Klein DF, Liebowitz MR (1998) Imipramine in the treatment of social phobia. *J Clin Psychopharmacol* 18: 132–135

41 Foa EB, Davidson J, Rothbaum BO (1995) Posttraumatic stress disorder. *In*: GO Gabbard (ed.): *Treatments of psychiatric disorders, second edition*. American Psychiatric Press, Washington D.C., 1499–1519

42 Davidson J (1992) Drug therapy of post-traumatic stress disorder. *Brit J Psychiat* 160: 309–314

43 American Psychiatric Association (1994) *Diagnostic and statistical manual of mental disorders, fourth edition (DSM-IV)*. American Psychiatric Association, Washington D.C., 417–423

44 Insel TR (1992) Toward a neuroanatomy of obsessive-compulsive disorder. *Arch Gen Psychiat* 49: 739–744

45 Pigott TA, Seay S (1997) Pharmacotherapy of obsessive compulsive disorder. *Int Rev Psychiat* 9: 133–147

46 Hoehn-Saric R, Harrison W, Clary C (1997) Obsessive-compulsive disorder with comorbid major depression: A comparison of sertraline and desipramine treatment. *Eur Neuropsychpharmacol* S 180

47 Greist JH, Jefferson JW, Kobak KA, Katzelnick DJ, Serlin RC (1995) Efficacy and tolerability of serotonin transport inhibitors in obsessive-compulsive disorder. *Arch Gen Psychiat* 52: 53–60

48 Barr LC, Goodman WK, Anand A, McDougle CJ, Price LH (1997) Addition of desipramine to serotonin reuptake inhibitors in treatment-resistant obsessive-compulsive disorder. *Amer J Psychiat* 154: 1293–1295

49 Fallon BA, Liebowitz MR, Campeas R, Schneier FR, Marshall R, Davies S, Goetz D, Klein DF (1998) Intravenous clomipramine for obsessive-compulsive disorder refractory to oral clomipramine: A placebo-controlled study. *Arch Gen Psychiat* 55: 918–924

50 Gittelman-Klein R, Klein DF (1973) School phobia: Diagnostic considerations in the light of imipramine effects. *J Nerv Ment Dis* 156: 199–215

51 Klein RG, Koplewicz HS, Kanner A (1992) Imipramine treatment of children with separation anxiety disorder. *J Amer Acad Child Adolesc Psychiat* 31: 1:21–28

52 Berney T, Kolvin I, Bhate SR, Garside RF, Jeans J, Kay B, Scarth L (1981) School phobia: A therapeutic trial with clomipramine and short-term outcome. *Brit J Psychiat* 138: 110–118

53 DeVeaugh-Geiss J, Moroz G, Biedermam J, Cantwell D, Fontaine R, Greist JH, Reichler R, Katz R, Landau P (1992) Clomipramine hydrochloride in childhood and adolescent obsessive compulsive disorder: A multicenter trial. *J Amer Acad Child Adolesc Psychiat* 31: 45–49

54 Geller B, Reising D, Leonard HL, Riddle MA (1999) Critical review of tricyclic antidepressant use in children and adolescents. *J Amer Acad Child Adolesc Psychiat* 38: 513–516

Anxiolytics
ed. by M. Briley and D. Nutt
© 2000 Birkhäuser Verlag/Switzerland

Monoamine oxidase inhibitors (including the newer reversible compounds)

Raimund Buller[1] and Karin M. Jorga[2]

[1] Quintiles, 3–5, rue Maurice Ravel, F-92594 Levallois-Perret, France
[2] F. Hoffmann-La Roche, Dept. of Clinical Pharmacology, Grenzachstrasse 124, CH-4070 Basel, Switzerland

Introduction

In the mid-1950s the chance finding of iproniazid's mood-elevating properties [1] led to the discovery that inhibition of monoamine oxidase (MAO) results in changes in cerebral function. Monoamine oxidase metabolizes and thus inactivates endogenous pressor amines (like serotonin and noradrenaline) as well as ingested amines absorbed from the gut (like tyramine). The therapeutic effect of MAOIs is supposed to be linked to an inhibition of the degradation of serotonin, noradrenaline and dopamine resulting in their increased availability. Among the various types of monoamine oxidases, those located in mitochondria, namely MAO-A and MAO-B, are of special interest for neuropsychiatry. Both enzymes are present in most tissues in the CNS but also in peripheral organs. MAO-A selectively deaminates serotonin and noradrenaline while benzylamines and phenythylamines are preferential substrates for MAO-B. In humans, dopamine is deaminated by both MAOs, hence the use of MAOIs in Parkinson's disease. First generation MAOIs are non-selective (inhibiting both enzymes) and irreversible, meaning that MAO is permanently inhibited by their action. MAO activity only resumed after treatment had been discontinued for several weeks, allowing new enzyme to be generated.

Initial open clinical trials illustrated iproniazid's antidepressant effects. However, double-blind, placebo-controlled studies were less convincing and led to controversies regarding the efficacy of MAOIs and their place in treatment of psychiatric disorders. Clear drawbacks of classical MAOIs also resulted from their side-effects (for review see [2]). During treatment the following adverse events are observed frequently: hypotension, increased body weight, sleepiness, agitation. Less often patients report sexual dysfunction, autonomic dysregulation or psychosis. Rare side-effects that have caused serious problems are hepatotoxicity (supposedly linked to hydrazine structure of the molecule) and hypertensive crises due to ingestion of tyramine-rich foodstuffs resulting in significant cardiovascular complications and even deaths. As a consequence many physicians avoid prescribing MAOIs. Even the removal of the more hepatotoxic compounds from the market and the development of a second generation of less toxic compounds like tranylcypromine (Parnate) or phenelzine (Nardil) as well as proper warnings for the patient to maintain a specified diet have not changed this trend. The use of MAOIs is still very limited and the drugs appear to be reserved for treatment-resistant or "atypical" cases of depression. As MAOIs seem to have some abuse potential (due to amphetamine-like properties) and may cause dependence, cautious use in individuals with substance abuse disorders is necessary.

Because of the potential for serious interaction a significant number of drugs are contraindicated for use in patients treated with MAOIs, including sympathomimetics, central stimulants, centrally acting antihypertensives and opoid analgesics. A combination of MAOIs with drugs that enhance serotonin (tricyclic antidepressants, serotonin reuptake inhibitors and pethidine), may lead to a "serotonin syndrome" [3], characterized by restlessness, shivering, tremor, increased body temperature, hyperreflexia, myoclonus, convulsions and even coma or death.

With the discovery of two isoenzymes of monoamine oxidases, types A and B, a search for compounds with selectivity was undertaken and resulted in the introduction of a third generation of irreversible inhibitors with relative specificity for the A (e.g. clorgyline) or B form (L-deprenyl). However, only the discovery of compounds that were both selective for MAO-A and reversible in their MAO inhibition (like moclobemide and brofaromine) caused a renewed interest in this psychopharmacological principle.

During the last 10–15 years compounds from the new group of reversible inhibitors of monoamine oxidase A (RIMA) like moclobemide, brofaromine, toloxatone and befloxatone have been tested extensively in depression and in other indications. However, so far only two have reached the market. Moclobemide (Aurorix) is licensed for the treatment of depression in more than 60 countries although not in the US (for details about the development history of moclobemide see Angst and colleagues [4], for a short overview on the use in depression see [5, 6]). Toloxatone (Humoryl) is currently marketed only in France and Italy. Main advantages of RIMAs are: benign side-effect profile, better tolerability, reduced toxicity, no dietary restrictions and safety in (mono-)overdose. However, rare fatalities have been reported for toloxatone [7] resulting from fulminant hepatitis and for moclobemide following mixed overdoses with serotonergic drugs, especially with co-administration of clomipramine [8].

MAOIs in the treatment of anxiety

Phenelzine is the most commonly used and most widely studied "classical" MAOI. Its efficacy in depressed patients has been subject to controversy since a number of trials produced inconclusive results namely when the doses used were rather low. Phenelzine performed best at higher doses and in outpatients likely to be suffering from depressive neurosis or "atypical" depression with features like increased appetite, overeating, sensitivity to rejection and prominent symptoms of anxiety [9]. In 1970, Kelly and co-workers [10] were interested in the efficacy in neurotic patients with phobias and presented a retrospective study of patients (including children) with agoraphobia, other phobias and panic attacks. All patients were treated with MAOIs either alone or in combination with benzodiazepines or tricyclics. The authors found a significant improvement in phobia ratings independent of the type of phobia, the previous personality or the presence or absence of depression. Treatment also had a dramatic effect on number and severity of panic attacks. Although the data came from a retrospective and uncontrolled study the results were superior to what had been previously observed during controlled trials. Tyrer et al. [11] confirmed the efficacy of phenelzine in phobic anxiety in a prospective placebo-controlled study. In a mixed sample of 32 patients with agoraphobia and/or social phobia phenelzine demonstrated significantly greater effects than placebo on general ratings and secondary phobias.

The usefulness of phenelzine in patients with patients with anxiety disorders was confirmed by Sheehan et al. [12] in a 12-week study of patients with "endogenous anxiety with phobia symptoms." This group suffered from panic attacks, sudden spells of somatic symptoms (e.g. dizzy spells, faintness, chest pain), and phobic fears (e.g. crowded places). Treatment with either phenelzine or imipramine was superior to placebo on measures of anxiety and depression. Patients in the phenelzine group had the best outcome and even showed significantly better results than imipramine patients with respect to avoidance behavior and work/social disability.

By 1980 there was good evidence that MAOIs were effective in patients with phobic anxiety and panic especially at higher doses and with sufficiently long duration of treatment. However, the samples were still not homogenous as the studies included varying proportions of subjects with different phobias (agoraphobia, social phobia, panic attacks). The new operationally defined classification of the DSM-III [13] (and succeeding revisions) provided the basis for trials in more narrowly defined groups of patients with specific anxiety disorders (like agoraphobia, panic disorder and social phobia).

Agoraphobia and panic disorder

Panic Disorder is a debilitating conditions characterized by sudden, unexpected attacks of anxiety which are often associated with physiological symptoms like tachycardia, dizziness, palpitations or with psychological symptoms like fear of dying and fear of loosing control. As a consequence patients often develop anticipatory anxiety and phobic avoidance which may lead to severe agoraphobia.

MAOIs in agoraphobia and panic disorder

Following the landmark study by Sheehan et al. [12], which mainly included subjects who would now be diagnosed as panic disorder with or without agoraphobia, only uncontrolled or open studies [14, 15] specifically tested the efficacy of classical MAOIs in this condition. The studies suggest that MAOIs may be superior to TCAs and that tranylcypromine may be as effective as phenelzine.

RIMAs in agoraphobia and panic disorder

Evidence for efficacy of reversible inhibitors of MAO-A (RIMA) comes from a number of controlled and uncontrolled studies. Berger et al. [16] compared the efficacy of moclobemide 100 mg/day to the efficacy of the drug at 400 mg/day in patients with panic disorder with or without agoraphobia in a trial over 9 weeks and found a moderate drug effect. Dilbaz et al. [17] conducted a double-blind study in 34 patients comparing moclobemide (up to 450 mg/day) and clomipramine (up to 150 mg/day). At the end of treatment both compounds had produced comparable results with 50 to 60% of the patients rated as "markedly improved" or "back to normal". Tiller et al. [18] reported on a comparative trial in 366 patients treated with moclobemide or fluoxetine for 8 weeks. Outcome was equivalent at the end of the study when more than 60% of the subjects (60.2% on moclobemide and 65.6% on fluoxetine) did not experience full panic attacks anymore. Based on the CGI rating 84% in the moclobemide group and 82% in the fluoxetine group were considered minimally, much or very much improved.

Two large placebo-controlled, fixed dose moclobemide studies with 300 or 600 mg/day have been conducted. Both studies showed similar findings: the percentage of patients considered responders (with a CGI rating of much or very much improved) was 51% for the subjects on 600 mg/day, 54% for 300 mg/day and 48% for placebo in one study, (protocol N13357, data on file F. Hoffmann-La Roche) and 60% (600 mg/day), 61% (300 mg/day) and 58% (placebo) in the other (protocol N13356, data on file F. Hoffmann-La Roche). Because of the high placebo response rate, the studies failed to demonstrate the efficacy of moclobemide. However, in a subgroup of more severely ill patients both trials found a markedly lower placebo response (33%–40%) and a markedly better drug response (48%–57% for 300 mg/day; 41%–62% for 600 mg/day). A third trial comparing the long-term efficacy of moclobemide 300 or 600 mg/day over 6 months (protocol 13358, data on file F. Hoffmann-La Roche) likewise failed to show efficacy due to a high placebo response rate (62%) and only numerically, but not statistically higher response rates for the two drug groups (65% for 300 mg/day; 67% for 600 mg/day). The outcomes of these three studies are in line with reports that in recent years clinical trial programs to test the efficacy of new potential treatments have faced an increasing problem of producing conclusive results. However, the small separation from placebo observed does not reflect the testing of weaker drugs since it applies not only to new compounds, but also to standard reference treatments [19].

Brofaromine, a RIMA for which the clinical development has been discontinued, was also tested in panic disorder in open-label and double-blind controlled trials. Garcia-Borreguero et al. [20] studied 14 inpatients with panic disorder treated with 150 mg of brofaromine and found a clear reduction of anxiety scores over time. Bakish et al. [21] compared brofaromine and clomipramine in an 8-week double-blind study with a total sample of 93 patients. Both groups showed similar improvement but the results have to be viewed in light of the fact that the study suffered from a high drop-out rate (63% for brofaromine, 49% for clomipramine) with the majority of premature terminations occurring during the first 2 weeks of the trial. In a 12-week double-blind placebo-controlled study van Vliet et al. [22] observed significant improvement with brofaromine (70% responders) but not with placebo (no responders). Features of anxiety, distress caused by panic attacks as well as agoraphobic avoidance improved with brofaromine. Most prominent side-effects were sleep disturbances and nausea. Brofaromine patients initially experienced a brief exacerbation of their anxiety during the first week of treatment. Similar biphasic treatment responses have been observed with serotonin reuptake inhibitors. The finding in this study may be explained by brofaromine's ability to also inhibit 5HT reuptake, which may play a role in the clinical profile of the drug [23].

The only other RIMA so far tested in panic disorder is toloxatone which was given for 7 days in a small single-blind placebo-controlled trial where the drug reduced the reactivity of panic patients to the inhalation of 35% CO_2. For befloxatone no clinical data on the efficacy in panic disorder have yet been published. However positive findings from animal models may predict efficacy in panic disorder [24].

In summary, although neither moclobemide nor any other compounds from this drug class have yet received a license for the treatment of panic disorder or agoraphobia the current evidence supports the efficacy of RIMA in these conditions. Their benign side-effect profile and the absence of negative effects on driving performance [25] suggests that they may be especially valuable in the treatment of outpatients.

Social phobia (social anxiety disorder)

The main diagnostic feature of social phobia (social anxiety disorder) is the patient's intense, irrational and persistent fear of being scrutinized or evaluated by others. Subjects anticipate that they will be subject to humiliation or ridicule. Dependent on the choice of criteria as many as 10% of the general population may suffer from social phobia [26]. Since the disorder starts during late adolescence or early adulthood many patients experience a lack in the development in their social skills which may result in significant maladjustment. Alcohol or tranquilizer when used in an attempt to self-medicate can be the cause of secondary abuse or dependence. Normal social discomfort even with some autonomic arousal is extremely common. Most people also tend to avoid situations where they would be the object of criticism or disapproval. However, this should not be confused with social phobia, a disorder which leads to severe impairment due to extreme fear of most situations where there is a possibility of being socially evaluated.

MAOIs in social phobia

Early studies in mixed populations of phobic patients and depressed subjects with "atypical" features (like sensitivity to rejection) already suggested that classical MAO-inhibitors may be effective in the treatment of social phobia. Supportive and definitive evidence was provided by a number of open and double-blind controlled studies in well-defined samples of patients with social phobia diagnosed according to operationalized criteria.

Liebowitz et al. [27] reported on phenelzine in a series of openly treated cases, where seven out of 11 subjects showed marked and four cases moderate improvement. When patients stopped treatment they experienced relapse. Versiani et al. [28] treated 32 patients with tranylcypromine and found supporting evidence for the efficacy of this MAOI in social phobia. Sixty-two percent of the sample showed marked improvement while 17% were moderately improved. A further open tranylcypromine study by Versiani et al. [29] in 81 patients also showed that the treatment resulted in significant improvement on measures of social phobia, mood and psychosocial impairment. Gelernter et al. [30] treated a total of 65 patients with social phobia with either alprazolam, phenelzine, placebo or cognitive behavior therapy (CBT). Subjects (even in the placebo group) received instructions for self-directed exposure to phobic stimuli and the study lacked a true "no-treatment" control group. All treatments were effective as patients in all groups showed significant changes on self-report measures and none was superior. Based on the social phobia subscale of the Fear Questionnaire patients were classified as responders if their score was below the population mean. On this basis phenelzine appeared to be most effective with 69% responders compared with 38% of the alprazolam-treated, 24% of the CBT-treated and 20% of the placebo patients. Liebowitz et al. [31] studied the efficacy of phenelzine and atenolol, a beta-blocker in comparison with placebo in a group of patients with social phobia. Eighty-five subjects were randomized and 74 completed at least 4 weeks of treatment. Among these, 64% (16/25) responded to phenelzine, 30% (7/23) to atenolol and 23% (6/26) to placebo. Including the randomized patients who dropped out before week 4 (intent to treat analysis) the responder rates were 55% for phenelzine, 25% for atenolol and 21% for placebo. Phenelzine, but not atenolol differed significantly from placebo with respect to response rates as well as on measures of social phobia and disability. A study similar in design to the previous trial but with phenelzine, moclobemide (instead of atenolol) and placebo was conducted by Versiani et al. [32]. The study is presented in detail in the following chapter on RIMAs in social phobia. Finally, Heimberg [33] reported on 133 patients from two sites who received 12 weeks of cognitive behavior group therapy (CBGT), phenelzine therapy, pill placebo administration, or educational-supportive group therapy (an attention-placebo treatment of equal credibility to CBGT). After 12 weeks, phenelzine therapy and CBGT led to superior response rates and greater change on dimensional measures of social phobia than did either control condition. However, response to phenelzine therapy was more evident after 6 weeks, and phenelzine therapy was also superior to CBGT after 12 weeks on some measures. There were few differences between sites, suggesting that these treatments can be efficacious at facilities with differing theoretical allegiances.

In summary, a number of studies support the efficacy of classical MAOIs like phenelzine or tranylcypromine in social phobia although the evidence is still based on rather small samples. Phenelzine is sometimes seen as "gold standard", "treatment of choice" or "first-line treatment" in social phobia. However, the total number of social phobia patients treated with MAOIs in controlled trials hardly exceeds 200, a database that would not be sufficiently large to apply for a product license. Since all studies to date have been carried out in a very small number of centers (single or dual center trials) and as no large multi-center trials have been conducted (where more impediments tend to exist to the demonstration of efficacy) it is difficult to assess the "true" effect sample size of classical MAOIs in this indication. In addition, an unfavorable safety profile and the need for dietary restrictions will probably continue to prevent the wide-spread use of MAOIs in this condition. As a result, the search for new treatments will continue.

RIMAs in social phobia

Moclobemide has been considered as a potential alternative to classical MAOIs and was investigated in a number of trials in social phobia. Versiani et al. [32] were the first to conduct a double-blind study comparing moclobemide with phenelzine and placebo. The target dose for moclobemide was 600 mg/day, for phenelzine 90 mg/day. After 16 weeks of treatment 19 out of 26 patients on phenelzine (73%), 14 out of 26 patients on moclobemide (54%) and only three out of 26 patients on placebo (12%) were nearly asymptomatic and therefore regarded as "responders". Side-effects were most common and more severe in the phenelzine group, including two adverse events (urinary retention and hypertensive crisis – both without sequalae) which led to discontinuation of treatment. Overall, 42% of the placebo patients (11/26), 82% of the moclobemide patients (21/26) and 92% of the patients receiving phenelzine (24/26) reported at least one adverse event. The first European trial, an open-label 12-week pilot study on moclobemide (dose range 300 to 600 mg/day) in social phobia by Bisserbe et al. [34] found a response rate of 48%. The drug improved phobic fears and avoidance, and was well-tolerated. The main side-effects produced were headache, insomnia and nervousness. The placebo-controlled moclobemide study by Schneier et al. [35] used a forced dose-escalation design with a target dose of 400 mg twice daily. Outcome in the treatment groups did not differ significantly as the sample response rates at week 8 were 7/40 (17.5%) for moclobemide and 5/37 (13.5%) for placebo. Although moclobemide was significantly superior on two of the primary outcome measures (the subscales for fear and avoidance of the Liebowitz Social Anxiety Scale) the overall treatment effect was rather modest. Drug-placebo differences in response rates were largest in severe or most-severe patients (23% for moclobemide, 0% for placebo). The most common side-effects with moclobemide were insomnia, fatigue, lightheadedness, excitement, and sedation. In a large (n = 506) placebo-controlled dose-response trial with five doses of moclobemide (75 mg, 150 mg, 300 mg, 600 mg and 900 mg daily) Noyes et al. [36] observed a significant linear regression of mean scores on the Liebowitz Scale (adjusted for baseline) over dose at weeks 8 and 12. However, for responder rates there was a trend in favor of higher doses only at 8 weeks but no difference in response to various doses of the drug at 12 weeks. Because of this lack of difference in response rates (33% for placebo, 35% for the highest moclobemide dose) the authors concluded that the trial had failed to demonstrate the efficacy of the drug. The results of this study are at variance with another large trial [37] which compared two doses of moclobemide (300 mg and 600 mg daily) with placebo in a sample of 578 subjects with social phobia. The authors report that the study showed consistent, reliable and clinically meaningful drug effects and indications of a dose-response relationship. At week 8 and 12 moclobemide at a dose of 600 mg per day was effective and statistically significantly different from placebo. Moclobemide treatment reduces symptoms of social phobia and impairment associated with the disorder. Response rates were 34% for placebo, 41% for the 300 mg and 47% for the 600 mg dose. Drug-placebo differences were largest in subjects with severe to most severe conditions (30.4% responders on placebo, 37.3% on 300 mg and 52.4% on 600 mg of moclobemide). The drug was well-tolerated; most common adverse events were insomnia, headaches, dizziness, and nausea. Long-term efficacy of moclobemide in social phobia is described in an open-label trial by Versiani et al. [38]; 101 patients were treated for up to 2 years. At the end of this period 58/99 (58.5%) were responders. Treatment was discontinued abruptly. Only seven patients were in remission while the majority reported a worsening of symptoms over the following 2 to 4 months. Treatment was re-initiated in 51 patients and symptoms gradually decreased again. Tolerability of moclobemide was very good with mainly mild adverse event. Most common side-effects were nausea, headache, insomnia, agitation and dizziness. The study supports the long-term safety and efficacy (maintenance of effects) over a treatment period of several years.

Evidence for the efficacy of brofaromine in social phobia comes from case studies and controlled trials. Garcia-Borreguero and Bronisch [39] treated a social phobia patient with brofaromine and observed a complete clinical remission after 4 weeks. No side-effects were reported. When the medication was discontinued the patient relapsed but became asymptomatic again when treatment was resumed. Bakish [40] presented the case of a patient with social phobia complicated by panic disorder. The subject was treated for a year and had a complete remission but relapsed after withdrawal. He experienced panic attacks again, developed agoraphobia and social phobia which did not respond to fluoxetine. Restarted again on brofaromine he became symptom-free. Van Vliet et al. [41] entered 30 social phobia patients in a 12-week study. Twelve out of the 15 patients on brofaromine (80%) but only two out of the 15 on placebo (14%) responded. The most prominent side-effects for brofaromine were insomnia, nausea, loss of appetite and weight loss. Fahlén et al. [42] conducted a similar study (n = 77) and observed a robust treatment effect with 78% responders in the brofaromine and only 23% responders in the placebo group. The drug improved social phobia symptoms and mood ratings. Patients on brofaromine showed further improvement during a 9-month follow-up treatment whereas 60% of the placebo responders had a relapse. Common side-effects were sleep disturbances, dry mouth and nausea. In a second paper on this study Fahlén [43] reported that maladaptive personality traits (like features of avoidant or dependent personality disorder) which are characteristic of social phobia also improved with brofaromine treatment. Lott et al. [44] reported results from a placebo-controlled multicenter brofaromine study in 102 patients. Brofaromine produced significantly greater effects than placebo in terms of measures of social phobia. However, since the mean final score on the social phobia measure was still in the clinical range, the authors conclude that the observed effect was modest. Fifty percent of patients on brofaromine were responders (rated "much improved" or "very much improved") *versus* only 19% on placebo. Side-effects more common in brofaromine included insomnia, dizziness, dry mouth, anorexia, tinnitus and tremor.

In summary, to date studies with RIMAs have been conducted in several hundred patients with social phobia and support the efficacy, safety and good tolerability of RIMAs in this indication. It is still an open question if RIMA produce more moderate effects than classical MAOIs as the two classes have not yet been compared in any large multicenter trials. Clearly, both drug classes, MAOIs and RIMAs, will have a place in the treatment of patients with social phobia, and in fact, moclobemide has already been awarded a license for that indication in some European countries. As social phobia is often treated successfully with behavior therapy more studies examining combinations of pharmacotherapy with psychological interventions should be conducted.

Post-traumatic stress disorder (PTSD)

PTSD is a complex psychiatric condition, defined by the presence of clinically significant reexperiencing, avoidance, numbing, and hyperarousal following the occurrence of an extremely stressful stimulus (trauma). Traumatic events, usually experienced with intense fear, terror, and helplessness include combat, criminal assault, rape, accidents or natural disasters. The condition is currently listed among the anxiety disorders presumably because it is accompanied by the concomitants of anxiety (e. g, insomnia, exaggerated startle response, and difficulty concentrating). However, it is possible for a patient to qualify for PTSD without any symptomatic anxiety.

MAOIs in PTSD

During the last 20 years, monoamine oxidase inhibitors have been frequently used in PTSD. A majority of early case reports and open trials support the usefulness of phenelzine in this population. Hogben and Cornfield treated five patients and saw decreases in flashbacks, nightmares and startling [45]. Walker reported on three subjects [46] and also observed decreased nightmares and flashbacks. In a series of eight cases Shen and Park [47] saw improvement but also sexual side-effects. In a series of six subjects treated by Milanes et al. [48] phenelzine improved sleep, anxiety, depressive and PTSD symptoms. Birkheimer et al. [49] used a variety of antidepressants in 15 PTSD patients. Phenelzine (three subjects) improved sleep and diminished depression and anxiety. Bleich et al. [50] likewise treated patients (n = 27) with various antidepressants; in two subjects on phenelzine the response was poor. Davidson et al. [51] observed positive effects of phenelzine in 11 subjects with marked improvement in flashbacks, intrusions and moderate improvement in sleep, startle, nightmares and guilt. At variance with this report is a study by Lerer et al. [52]. Based on the treatment of 25 inpatients they saw only modest effects of phenelzine. The study by Shetatzky et al. [53] which also did not detect a difference between phenelzine and placebo suffered from insufficient power due to the small sample size (n = 13). Frank et al. [54] in a comparison between imipramine, phenelzine and placebo (n = 34) reported greater reduction of PTSD symptoms with the MAOI.

Most pharmacological studies were conducted in combat veterans and therefore findings cannot necessarily be generalized to other PTSD populations. The adverse event profile of MAOIs has significantly limited their utility for the treatment of PTSD. MAOIs are especially problematic in subjects who continue their substance abuse as the consequences of noncompliance with the tyramine-free diet are potentially serious.

RIMA in PTSD

Only three studies with RIMAS in PTSD have been reported so far. In the first [55], an open trial with a target dose of 600 mg of moclobemide, 20 subjects were treated for up to 12 weeks. The majority of patients (61%) showed PTSD syndromal recovery. Improvement was seen on a majority of PTSD symptoms, measures of anxiety, depression and social disability. Adverse events were mild and included headache, gastrointestinal complaints and loss of appetite.

Brofaromine was then tested in large multicenter placebo-controlled trial in 118 patients with PTSD [56]. Both groups showed significant improvement over time. However there were no significant difference between the treatments. A second multicenter trial reported by Katz et al. [57] comparing brofaromine and placebo in 45 subjects showed significant improvement during the trial but likewise failed to show statistically significant differences between the treatment groups.

In summary, the findings concerning RIMAs in PTSD are inconclusive. RIMAs are clearly well-tolerated in this population but it is unclear if they will be of therapeutic benefit.

References

1 Kline NS (1970) Monoamine oxidase inhibitors. *In*: FG Ayd, B Blackwell (eds): *Discoveries in biological psychiatry*. Lippincott, Philadelphia, 194–204
2 Livingston MG, Livingston HM (1996) Monoamine oxidase inhibitors. An update on drug interactions. *Drug Safety* 14: 219–227
3 Sternbach H (1991) Serotonin syndrome. *Amer J of Psychiat* 148: 705–713
4 Angst J, Amrein R, Stabl M (1996) Moclobemide: a paradigm of research in clinical psychopharmacology. *Int Clin Psychopharmacol* 11 (suppl. 3): 3–7
5 Freeman H (1993) Moclobemide. *Lancet* 342: 1528–1532
6 Fulton B, Benfield (1996) Moclobemide. An update of its pharmacological properties and therapeutic use. *Drugs* 52: 450–474
7 Pateron D, Babany G, Hadengue A, Delafosse B, Degott C, Sylvain C, Larrey D, Benhamou JP (1990) Hépatites fulminantes mortelles chez deux femmes prenant de la toloxatone (Humoryl) *Gastroenterol Clin Biol* 14: 504–506
8 Neuvonen PJ, Pohjola-Sintonen S, Tacke U, Vuori E (1993) Five fatal cases of serotonin syndrome after moclobemide-citalopram or moclobemide-clomipramine overdoses. *Lancet* 342: 1419
9 Robinson DS, Nies A, Ravaris CL, Lamborn KR (1973) The monoamine oxidase inhibitor, phenelzine, in the treatment of depressive-anxiety states. *Arch Gen Psychiat* 29: 407–413
10 Kelly D, Guirguis W, Frommer E, Mitchell-Heggs N, Sargant W (1970) Treatment of phobic states with antidepressants. *Brit J Psychiat* 116: 387–398
11 Tyrer P, Candy J, Kelly D (1973) A study of the clinical effects of phenelzine and placebo in the treatment of phobic anxiety. *Psychopharmacologia* 32: 237–254
12 Sheehan DV, Ballenger J, Jacobsen G (1980) Treatment of endogenous anxiety with phobic, hysterical, and hypochondriacal symptoms *Arch Gen Psychiat* 37: 51–59
13 American Psychiatric Association (1980) *Diagnostic and statistical manual of mental disorders, third edition*. APA, Washington, D.C.
14 Ballenger JC, Howell EF, Laraia M et al (1987) Comparison of four medicines in panic disorder. *Paper presented at the annual meeting of the American Psychiatric Association*, Chicago
15 Versiani M, Costa e Silva JA, Klerman GL (1987) Treatment of panic disorder with alprazolam, clomipramine, imipramine, tranylcypromine or placebo. *Paper presented at the annual meeting of*

the American College of Neuropsychopharmacology. San Juan, Puerto Rico

16 Berger P, Amering M, Dantendorfer K, Alf C, Kutzer M, Katschnig H (1991) Moclobemide in Panic Disorder. *(Abstract) 5th World Congress of Biological Psychiatry,* Florence, Italy

17 Dilbaz N, Arihan AG (1993) Reversible MAO Inhibitor in the treatment of panic disorder. *Paper presented at the 9th World Congress of Psychiatry,* Rio de Janiero, Brazil

18 Tiller JWG, Bouwer C, Behnke K (1997) Moclobemide for anxiety disorders: a focus on moclobemide for panic disorder. *Int Clin Psychopharmacol* 12 (suppl 69) S27–S30

19 Montgomery SA (1999) The failure of placebo-controlled studies. *Eur Neuropsychopharmacol* 9: 271–276

20 Garcia-Borreguero D, Lauer CJ, Özdaglar A, Wiedemann K, Holsboer F, Krieg JC (1992) Brofaromine in panic disorder: a pilot study with a new reversible inhibitor of monoamine oxidase A. *Pharmacopsychiatry* 25: 261–264

21 Bakish D, Saxena BM, Bowen R, D'Souza J (1993) Reversible monoamine oxidase-A inhibitors in panic disorder. *Clin Neuropsychopharmacol* 16 (suppl 2) S77–S82

22 Van Vliet IM, Westenberg HGM, Den Boer JA (1993) MAO inhibitors in panic disorder: clinical effects of treatment with brofaromine. *Psychopharmacology* 112.483–489

23 Waldmeier PC, Graf T, Germer M, Feldtrauer JJ, Howald H (1993) Serotonin uptake inhibition by monoamine oxidase inhibitor brofaromine *Biol Psychiat* 33: 373–379

24 Griebel G, Perrault G, Sanger DJ (1997) Behavioural profiles of the reversible monoamine-oxidase-A inhibitors befloxatone and moclobemide in an experimental model for screening anxiolytic and anti-panic drugs. *Psychopharmacology* 131: 180–186

25 Ramaekers JG, van Veggel LMA, O'Hanlon JF (1994) A cross-study comparison of the effects of moclobemide and brofaromine on the actual driving performance and estimated sleep. *Clin Neuropharmacol* 17 (suppl 1) S9–S18

26 Degonda M, Angst J (1993) The Zurich study. XX. Social phobia and agoraphobia. *Eur Arch Psychiat Clin Neurosci* 243: 95–102

27 Liebowitz MR, Fyer AJ, Gorman JM, Campeas R, Levin A (1986) Phenelzine in social phobia. *J Clin Psychopharmacol* 6: 93–98

28 Versiani M, Mundim FD, Nardi AE, Liebowitz MR (1988) Tranylcypromine in social phobia. *J Clin Psychopharmacol* 8: 279–283

29 Versiani M, Nardi AE, Mundim FD (1989) Fobia social. *J Brasileiro Psiquiatria* 38: 251–263

30 Gelernter CS, Uhde TW, Cimbolic P, Arnkoff DB, Vittone BJ, Tancer ME, Bartko JJ (1991) Cognitive-behavioral and pharmacological treatments of social phobia. *Arch Gen Psychiat* 48: 938–945

31 Liebowitz MR, Schneier F, Campeas R, Hollander E, Hatterer J, Fyer A, Gorman J, Papp L, Davies S, Gully R, Klein DF (1992) Phenelzine vs atenolol in social phobia. A placebo-controlled comparison. *Arch Gen Psychiat* 49: 290–300

32 Versiani M, Nardi AE, Mundim FD, Alves AB, Liebowitz MR, Amrein R (1992) Pharmacotherapy of social phobia. *Brit J Psychiat* 161: 353–360

33 Heimberg RG, Liebowitz MR, Hope DA, Schneier FR, Holt CS, Welkowitz LA, Juster HR, Campeas R, Bruch MA, Cloitre M, Fallon B, Klein DF (1998) Cognitive behavioral group therapy vs phenelzine therapy for social phobia: 12-week outcome. *Arch Gen Psychiat* 55: 1133–1141

34 Bisserbe JC, Lépine JP, GRP group (1994) Moclobemide in social phobia: a pilot open study. *Clin Neuropharmacol* 17 (suppl 1): S88–S94

35 Schneier FR, Goetz D, Campeas R, Fallon B, Marshall R, Liebowitz MR (1998) Placebo-controlled trial of moclobemide in social phobia. *Brit J Psychiat* 172: 70–77

36 Noyes R, Moroz G, Davidson JRT, Liebowitz MR, Davidson A, Siegel J, Bell J, Cain JW, Curlik SM, Kent TA et al (1997) Moclobemide in social phobia: a controlled dose-response trial. *J Clin Psychopharmacol* 17: 247–254

37 International Multicenter Clinical Trial Group on Moclobemide in Social Phobia (1997) Moclobemide in social phobia. *Eur Arch Psychiat Clin Neurosci* 247: 71–80

38 Versiani M, Nardi AE, Mundim FD, Pinto S, Saboya E, Kovacs R (1996) The long-term treatment of social phobia with moclobemide. *Int Clin Psychopharmacol* 11 (suppl 3): 83–88

39 Bakish D (1994) The use of the reversible monoamine oxidase-A inhibitor brofaromine in social phobia complicated by panic disorder with or without agoraphobia. *J Clin Psychopharmacol* 14: 74–75

40 Garcia-Borreguero D, Bronisch T (1992) Improvement of social phobic symptoms after treatment with brofaromine, a reversible and selective inhibitor of MAO-A. *Eur Psychiat* 7: 93–94

41 Van Vliet IM, den Boer JA, Westenberg HGM (1992) Psychopharmacological treatment of social phobia: clinical and biochemical effects of brofaromine, a selective MAO-A inhibitor. *Eur Neuropsychopharmacol* 2: 21–29

42 Fahlén T, Nilsson HL, Borg K, Humble M, Pauli U (1995) Social phobia: the clinical efficacy and tolerability of the monoamine oxidase-A and serotonin uptake inhibitor brofaromine. *Acta Psychiat Scand* 92: 351–358

43 Fahlén T (1995) Personality traits in social phobia, II: changes during treatment. *J Clin Psychiat* 56: 569–573

44 Lott M, Greist J, Jefferson JW, Kobak KA, Katzelnick DJ, Katz RJ, Schaettle SC (1997) Brofaromine for social phobia: a multicenter, placebo-controlled, double-blind study. *J Clin Psychopharmacol* 17: 255–260

45 Hogben GL, Cornfield RB (1981) Treatment of traumatic war neuroses with phenelzine. *Arch Gen Psychiat* 38: 440–445

46 Walker JI (1982) Chemotherapy of traumatic war stress. *Milit Med* 147: 1029–1033

47 Shen WW, Park S (1983) The use of monoamine oxidase inhibitors in the treatment of traumatic war neurosis. *Milit Med* 148: 430–431

48 Milanes FJ, Mack CN, Dennison J et al (1984) Phenelzine treatment of post-Vietnam stress syndrome. *VA Practitioner* June: 40–49

49 Birkheimer LJ, DeVane CL, Muniz CE (1985) Posttraumatic stress disorder: characteristics and pharmacological response in the veteran population. *Compr Psychiat* 26: 304–310

50 Bleich A, Siegel B, Garb R (1986) Post-traumatic stress disorder following combat exposure: clinical features and psychopharmacological treatment. *Brit J Psychiat* 149: 365–369

51 Davidson JRT, Walker JI, Kilts C (1987) A pilot study of phenelzine in the treatment of post-traumatic stress disorder. *Brit J Psychiat* 150: 252–255

52 Lerer B, Bleich A, Kotler M, Garb R, Hertzberg M, Levin B (1987) Posttraumatic stress disorder in Israeli combat veterans: effects of phenelzine treatment. *Arch Gen Psychiat* 44: 976–981

53 Shestatzky M, Greenberg D, Lerer B (1988) A controlled trial of phenelzine in posttraumatic stress disorder. *Psychiat Res* 24: 149–155

54 Frank JB, Kosten TR, Giller Jr EL, Dan E (1988) A randomized clinical trial of phenelzine and imipramine for posttraumatic stress disorder. *Amer J Psychiat* 145: 1289–1291

55 Neal LA, Shapland W, Fox C (1997) An open trial of moclobemide in the treatment of post-traumatic stress disorder. *Int Clin Psychopharmacol* 12: 231–237

56 Baker DG, Diamond BI, Gillette G, Hamner M, Katzelnick D, Keller T, Mellman TA, Pontius E, Rosenthal M, Tucker et al (1995) A double-blind, randomized, placebo-controlled, multi-center study of brofaromine in the treatment of post-traumatic stress disorder. *Psychopharmacology* 122: 386–389

57 Katz RJ, Lott MH, Arbus P, Crocq L, Herlobsen P, Lingjaerde O, Lopez G, Loughrey GC, Macfarlane DJ, McIvor R et al. (1994/1995) Pharmacotherapy of post-traumatic stress disorder with a novel psychotropic. *Anxiety* 1: 169–174

Anxiolytics
ed. by M. Briley and D. Nutt
© 2000 Birkhäuser Verlag/Switzerland

Selective serotonin re-uptake inhibitors in anxiety disorders: room for improvement

David S. Baldwin[1] and Jon Birtwistle[2]

[1] *Mental Health Group, Faculty of Medicine, Health and Biological Sciences, University of
Southampton, UK*
[2] *Primary Medical Care Group, Faculty of Medicine, Health and Biological Sciences, University of
Southampton, UK*

Introduction

As a group, the SSRIs have been found efficacious in double-blind placebo-controlled studies across a range of depressive disorders, both in short-term and long-term treatment. The efficacy of SSRIs is similar to that of tricyclic anti-depressants (TCAs) in patients with major depression, apart from in the sub-group of hospitalised in-patients, where TCAs are marginally, but significantly, more effective [1]. In randomised controlled trials, the tolerability of SSRIs is better than that of TCAs, there being significantly fewer drop-outs from treatment because of adverse effects, but the magnitude of this difference is rather small [2]. SSRIs are clearly safer than most TCAs, when taken in over-dose; and being less sedative, are less likely to interfere with many aspects of everyday life. For these reasons, the SSRIs have gained widespread acceptance in the treatment of depression, both in primary and secondary care settings.

The early concern that SSRIs might worsen anxiety or agitation in some depressed patients is probably unfounded, as a number of pooled analyses have suggested that the presence of higher anxiety scores at baseline does not preclude depressed patients from making a satisfactory response to treatment with SSRIs (for example, see [3]). This observation, together with the findings of abnormalities of serotonergic function in pre-clinical studies in animal models, and in biological investigations in humans, naturally led to the evaluation of SSRIs as potential treatments for anxiety disorders. Numerous double-blind, placebo-controlled studies of SSRIs in panic disorder, obsessive-compulsive disorder, social phobia and post-traumatic stress disorder have been conducted, many of which have found that SSRIs are as effective as other anxiolytic treatments, but sometimes with greater overall tolerability.

Quite why SSRIs are efficacious in the treatment of such a broad range of anxiety disorders is unknown. Whilst a relationship between serotonin and anxiety has long been postulated, the pathophysiological mechanisms and sites of possible abnormality have never been clear [4]. Pre-clinical studies indicate that the relationship between 5-HT and animal models of anxiety is complex, with different brain regions being implicated in differing aspects of anxiety [5]. The periaqueductal grey matter may be particularly involved in panic, and the amygdala in anticipatory anxiety and conditioned avoidance [6]. In human volunteers, acute neuroendocrine challenge tests in panic disorder and obsessive-compulsive disorder have produced rather inconsistent results [5, 7]. Finally, treatment studies in humans suggest that more selective serotonergic agents (such as the 5-HT2 antagonist ritanserin or the 5-HT3 antagonist ondansetron) are ineffective in anxiety, in contrast to the SSRIs [8].

In order to examine the efficacy of SSRIs in the treatment of the common anxiety disorders, the relevant scientific literature was "captured" by performing a computerized search of the Medline Express and Embase data sources for the period from January 1985 to June 1999. The search terms included each of the six SSRIs that have become available to clinicians (i.e. citalopram, fluoxetine, fluvoxamine, paroxetine, sertraline and zimelidine), together with appropriate free text words (anxiety, panic, ocd, obsessive, compulsive, disorder, obsessive compulsive disorder, social, phobia, social phobia, social anxiety, gad, generalised, anxiety, generalised anxiety, post, traumatic, stress, post traumatic stress and ptsd). The relevant psychopharmacological treatment studies were identified by using the free text words "double-blind-method" and "randomised-controlled-trials". Using this method, a total of 198 papers were identified by consulting Medline Express, and a total of 148 by consulting Embase. If necessary, further references were obtained by examining the bibliography sections of the papers identified by the computer search. In addition, the search was extended to include a number of recent treatment studies with SSRIs that had only been published in abstract form.

Panic disorder

Zimelidine

The first randomised controlled trial of an SSRI in panic disorder involved treatment with either zimelidine, imipramine or placebo [9]. In a group of 44 patients, zimelidine was found to be more efficacious than either placebo or imipramine. Unfortunately, treatment with zimelidine was associated with the development of a disorder akin to Guillain-Barre syndrome, and it was therefore withdrawn from clinical use [10]

Fluvoxamine

Treatment with fluvoxamine has been evaluated in a number of placebo-controlled and comparator-controlled treatment studies. Through a series of elegant investigations conducted by researchers in Utrecht, some of the early controlled trials with fluvoxamine were able to clarify the role of serotonin in the pathophysiology of panic disorder. The first of these studies involved treatment of 50 patients with either fluvoxamine or clomipramine [11]. Both drugs were found to be efficacious, with reductions in both anxiety and depressive symptoms – at the end of the study, 15 of the 26 clomipramine-treated and 14 of the 24 fluvoxamine-treated patients were free from symptoms. The authors followed this study with a second randomised controlled trial, involving treatment with either fluvoxamine or maprotiline, a noradrenaline re-uptake inhibitor [12]. Fluvoxamine treatment was associated with a reduction in anxiety and depressive symptoms and a decrease in the number of panic attacks, whereas maprotiline had little effect on measures of anxiety. At the end of the study, 10 of the 20 patients treated with fluvoxamine had improved substantially, compared to only five of 24 patients who received maprotiline. In a third study, the effects of fluvoxamine were then compared to treatment with the post-synaptic 5-HT2 receptor blocker ritanserin, to see whether 5-HT2 receptor function is abnormal in patients with panic disorder [13]. When compared to placebo or ritanserin, only fluvoxamine was found to be efficacious, with a significant reduction in the number of panic attacks, and significant improvements in anxiety and depressive symptoms and avoidance behaviour.

A series of subsequent placebo-controlled studies have provided further evidence for the efficacy of fluvoxamine in panic disorder. In an eight-week study involving 50 patients, treatment with fluvoxamine (mean daily dose at endpoint, 206.8 mg) was associated with a reduction in panic attacks from the third week, and with improvements in anxiety and depressive symptoms from the sixth week [14]. At the end of the study, 61% of the fluvoxamine group were free of panic attacks, compared to only 22% of those who received placebo. However, the panic attacks that remained were no less severe [14]. In another placebo-controlled trial that included 188 patients, fluvoxamine was also found to be significantly more efficacious than placebo, with greater reductions in panic attack frequency and Clinical Anxiety Scale scores, becoming apparent from the second week of treatment [15]. These two studies are partly supported by the findings of a third placebo-controlled investigation in 46 patients [16], in which fluvoxamine produced a significantly greater reduction in the number of limited symptom attacks (but not full panic attacks).

Treatment of panic disorder with fluvoxamine has also been compared to treatment with imipramine [17, 18] or brofaromine [19]. In an eight-week multi-centre double-blind placebo-controlled trial involving 148 patients, fluvoxamine (mean daily dose at endpoint, 171.4 mg) was found to be less effective than imipramine (164.7 mg) [17]. This finding may have been partly due to the chance observation that patients in the placebo group had significantly fewer panic attacks at baseline than those in the two active treatment groups: a further analysis, using the data from only one centre, was able to reveal evidence for the efficacy of both imipramine and fluvoxamine [18]. In a study of

30 patients, treated with either fluvoxamine (daily dose, 150 mg) or the reversible monoamine oxidase inhibitor brofaromine, both treatments were found efficacious. The participating patients described themselves as much or very much improved (93% brofaromine, 87% fluvoxamine), although only a minority had reductions of 50% or more on the Hamilton Anxiety Scale [19].

Fluvoxamine has also been compared to cognitive therapy, in two placebo-controlled studies [20, 21]. In the first, fluvoxamine was found to be superior to both cognitive therapy and placebo – by the end of an eight-week study involving 75 patients, 90% of the fluvoxamine group had achieved moderate to marked improvement, compared to 50% in the cognitive therapy group, and 39% in those receiving placebo. In the fluvoxamine group, 81% became free of panic attacks, this figure being less with cognitive therapy (53%) or place-bo (29%). This advantage for fluvoxamine may have been partly due to an earlier onset of action. Depressive symptoms improved in parallel with changes in panic attacks and anxiety symptoms [22]. A subsequent report from the same group showed that treatment with cognitive therapy produced more beneficial changes in "abnormal personality traits", which were found to be relatively resistant to fluvoxamine or placebo [23]. In the second placebo-controlled study [21], which included 190 primary care patients and lasted 13 weeks, cognitive behaviour therapy was found to be more effective than fluvoxamine; the greatest improvements were seen with cognitive behaviour therapy and fluvoxamine in combination [21, 24].

Fluoxetine

For a drug that has gained such widespread acceptance in the treatment of depression, it is surprising that fluoxetine has been studied so infrequently in panic disorder. The efficacy of fluoxetine has been evaluated in just one placebo-controlled trial, comprising acute and continuation phases [25, 26]. The relative efficacy of treatment with fluoxetine has also been evaluated in a "pilot trial", with desipramine as the comparator compound [27].

In the acute phase of the placebo-controlled study, 243 panic disorder patients were randomised to receive either placebo or one of two daily doses (10 mg or 20 mg) of fluoxetine for 10 weeks [25]. Treatment with fluoxetine was associated with greater reductions in panic attack frequency, phobic symptoms and functional impairment. These changes were most noticeable with the higher dose of fluoxetine; the 10 mg daily dose was not significantly different to placebo on measures of anxiety symptoms, work impairment, anticipatory anxiety or overall functioning, although the lower dose was linked to a significant reduction in panic attack frequency. In the continuation phase [26], 88 patients who had responded to fluoxetine were randomly allocated to either continue with fluoxetine, or to switch to placebo, both groups being followed up over the subsequent 24 weeks. Those continuing with active treatment showed a significant improvement in panic attack frequency and measures of phobic avoidance, whereas those switched to placebo had significantly worsened anxiety and depressive symptoms.

Paroxetine

The efficacy of paroxetine in the short-term and long-term treatment of patients with panic disorder has been investigated in a series of placebo-controlled multi-centre trials in Europe and America, some of which have also included a comparator psychotropic drug.

In the first study [28], 120 patients with panic disorder received either a flexible dose of paroxetine or placebo, in addition to cognitive behaviour therapy. There was a significantly greater reduction in panic attack frequency in patients receiving paroxetine, compared to those taking placebo, this difference being observable from the sixth week of treatment. However, the majority (64%) of patients who responded to paroxetine were still experiencing panic attacks at the end of the study. The optimal dosage of paroxetine in the acute treatment of panic disorder is around 40 mg/day, this having been established in two placebo-controlled studies ([29], Data on file, SmithKline Beecham Pharmaceuticals). In the first of these, 425 patients received either placebo or 10, 20 or 40 mg/day of paroxetine; only the 40 mg daily dose was significantly more efficacious than placebo, 86% of patients becoming free of panic attacks at this dosage [29].

The relative efficacy of paroxetine, compared to other psychotropic drugs, has been examined in a series of studies. In one investigation [30], 367 patients were randomised to receive placebo, paroxetine (daily dose, 20–60 mg) or clomipramine (daily dose, 50–150 mg). More patients in the group treated with paroxetine experienced a complete resolution of panic attacks by the end of the 12-week study, with evidence of a significantly earlier onset of action with paroxetine, compared to treatment with clomipramine. Those patients who had completed this acute phase investigation satisfactorily could then continue with treatment for a further 36 weeks. Panic attacks in the active treatment groups continued to decrease during the maintenance study. At the end of the continuation period, 85% of paroxetine-treated patients were free from panic attacks, compared to 72% of those allocated to clomipramine, and 59% in those receiving placebo [31]. However, a further comparator-controlled study produced less encouraging results (Data on file, SmithKline Beecham Pharmaceuticals). When compared to treatment with placebo or alprazolam, there was no advantage for paroxetine, probably because of unusually high response rates among patients receiving placebo.

Evidence for the long-term efficacy of paroxetine comes from the continuation treatment study involving clomipramine [31], together with an investigation which employed a "relapse prevention" design. A total of 175 patients who had responded to acute treatment were randomly allocated to either continue with paroxetine, or to switch to placebo. Only 5% of patients who continued with paroxetine relapsed, compared to 30% in those patients switched to placebo [32].

Sertraline

The results of several large double-blind placebo-controlled studies of sertraline in the treatment of panic disorder have been published [33–35]. In two studies of identical design, which together included 342 patients with panic disorder [33, 34], sertraline (50–200 mg per day) was found to be significantly more effective than placebo in reducing the "panic attack burden" (a product of the number and severity of panic attacks), from the second week of treatment. Significantly more patients became free of panic attacks on sertraline (59.3%) than on placebo (46.3%). In addition, there were greater improvements with sertraline in quality-of-life measures, including items relating to mood, work, social, family and leisure activities, and in overall satisfaction with life. In one study [34] adverse events were as frequent with sertraline and placebo; in the other [33] significantly more patients stopped treatment with sertraline because of adverse experiences.

In a third double-blind, placebo-controlled study, 178 patients received fixed daily doses of sertraline (50, 100 or 200 mg) for 12 weeks [35]. Sertraline was found to be superior in reducing the number of panic attacks and limited symptom attacks, and in improving anxiety symptoms. Although there were advantages for sertraline on scores on the Clinical Global Impression scale earlier in the study, there was no difference from placebo at the end of treatment. The number of patients dropping out from the study were similar for active and placebo treatment, but significantly more patients discontinued sertraline because of adverse events (mainly dry mouth and delayed ejaculation). The authors concluded that there was no advantage in increasing the dose of sertraline above 50 mg per day [35].

The relative efficacy of sertraline, compared to other treatments for panic disorder, is uncertain. A double-blind placebo-controlled study that compared sertraline to imipramine, yet to be published, found no advantage for active treatment over placebo, probably because of high placebo response rates (Data on file, Pfizer Inc.).

Citalopram

There are relatively few placebo-controlled studies of citalopram in panic disorder, although it has been available in some European countries for many years. In an 8-week treatment study of 475 patients with panic disorder, three differing doses of citalopram were compared to placebo and clomipramine [36]. The lowest daily dose of citalopram (10–15 mg) was not different to placebo, but the higher doses (20–30 mg, and 40–60 mg) were associated with significantly greater reductions in the frequency of panic attacks and measures of anxiety and depressive symptoms. Those patients who completed the acute study, and who were expected to benefit from longer-term treatment, could then be included in a second, one-year double-blind continuation study [37]. In the 279 patients who entered this second phase of treatment, the effects of the lowest dose of citalopram were again found to be no different to those of placebo. Those patients who received the higher doses of citalopram, or who continued with clomipramine, had the best chances of responding over the 12-month period. There were few differences in tolerability between citalopram and clomipramine. Although patients who received the higher doses of citalopram made similar improvements to those who were treated with clomipramine, the daily dose of clomipramine in both phases of treatment was rather low (60–90 mg) and further studies are probably required to establish the relative efficacy of citalopram.

Synthesis

Most, but not all, of the double-blind placebo-controlled studies of SSRIs in the acute and continuation treatment of patients with panic disorder have found evidence for the efficacy of active treatment. However, the magnitude of improvement during treatment is variable – the proportion of patients becoming free from panic attacks ranges from 36% [28] to 86% [29], highest response rates with SSRIs being seen in those studies which also show greater improvements on placebo [38]. Similar variation is seen in measures of global anxiety [38].

Differences in study design do not allow exact comparison of the efficacy of different SSRIs, there being a persistent need for head-to-head comparisons. Although a meta-analysis of 27 placebo-controlled randomised controlled trials concluded that treatment with SSRIs was more effective than treatment with either imipramine or alprazolam [39], this was published in 1995 and is therefore now out of date. The relative side-effect burden with differing treatments is also unclear, although a recent systematic overview suggests that SSRIs are better tolerated than other pharmacological treatments [40]. The relative efficacy of SSRIs and psychological approaches remains unclear, although there is some evidence that combination treatment may produce optimal results [21].

Obsessive-compulsive disorder

Fluvoxamine

Fluvoxamine was the first SSRI to be studied in patients with obsessive-compulsive disorder (OCD), a series of placebo-controlled and comparator-controlled studies showing that fluvoxamine is efficacious in short-term treatment. The potential efficacy of fluvoxamine in long-term treatment has not been studied extensively, although one study suggests that the dosage of fluvoxamine can be reduced in continuation therapy, after earlier response to acute treatment [41].

An early double-blind, placebo-controlled, cross-over study of fluvoxamine, involving just 20 patients, found that fluvoxamine treatment was associated with significantly greater reductions in obsessive-compulsive, anxiety and depressive symptoms. Response to fluvoxamine was not dependent upon the presence of co-existing depressive symptoms [42]. This observation was supported by the findings of a subsequent study of 42 patients with OCD [43], in which fluvoxamine was significantly more effective than placebo on all measures of obsessive-compulsive symptoms, in both depressed and non-depressed patients. However, a third placebo-controlled study of fluvoxamine and exposure therapy in 60 patients, found that the presence of depression influenced the effects of fluvoxamine on compulsive rituals, although study design features make interpretation difficult [44]. A one-year follow-up of the patients who had participated in this study suggested that exposure therapy in acute treatment reduced the need for antidepressant drugs [45].

These early investigations are supported by the findings of two more recent larger studies [46, 47]. In the first, there was a significantly greater improvement in the Clinical Global Impression scale, and the Y-BOCS and NIMH-OC scales during treatment with fluvoxamine, from the fourth and the sixth weeks of treatment, respectively [46]. In the second, 160 patients with OCD received placebo or flexible daily doses of fluvoxamine (100–300 mg) for 10 weeks. Treatment with fluvoxamine was significantly more effective than placebo, but only 33.3% of patients who received fluvoxamine were considered "responders" at the end of the study, compared to 9.0% of those who had received placebo, emphasizing the rather small changes that often occur during short-term treatment studies in patients with OCD [47].

The relative efficacy of fluvoxamine in OCD, compared to other treatment approaches has also been studied. For example, a series of studies have compared the anti-obsessional effects of fluvoxamine to those of clomipramine. In a 10-week, double-blind treatment study involving 65 patients with OCD, fluvoxamine (flexible daily dose, 100–250 mg) was similar in efficacy to clomipramine. There were no difference in overall tolerability, there being more anticholinergic side-effects and sexual dysfunction with clomipramine, and more headache and insomnia with fluvoxamine [48]. A second study in 79 patients also found that fluvoxamine and clomipramine were similarly efficacious, overall response rates being 56% with fluvoxamine and 54% with clomipramine [49]. Similar overall findings were seen in a third comparative study against clomipramine, although clomipramine had an earlier onset of action [50]. The results of further studies of fluvoxamine and behaviour therapy [51, 52] indicate that the addition of fluvoxamine may enhance the efficacy of behaviour therapy, particularly in patients with marked obsessions [51], although this has not been replicated [52].

Fluoxetine

Several double-blind, placebo-controlled studies have examined the efficacy of fluoxetine in the short-term and long-term treatment of OCD, both in adults [53, 54] and in children and adolescents [55].

In a European double-blind multi-centre study, 217 patients with OCD were randomised to receive either placebo or one of three fixed daily doses of fluoxetine (20, 40 or 60 mg) for 8 weeks [53]. There was a statistically significant advantage for fluoxetine treatment in the overall responder rates, as defined by changes on both the Y-BOCS scale and Clinical Global Impression scale, although the magnitude of the treatment effect was marginal on other outcome measures. The highest dose of fluoxetine was associated with the highest response rate.

These observations are supported by the findings of two North American multi-centre studies, which followed identical treatment protocols and were subject to a pooled analysis [55]. 355 patients received either placebo or 20, 40 or 60 mg of fluoxetine per day, for 13 weeks. Again, fluoxetine was found to be superior to placebo on a variety of outcome measures, this advantage for fluoxetine being apparent from the fifth week of treatment. There was some suggestion that the highest dose was the most efficacious, this being supported by the findings of a subsequent continuation phase study [54]. In this, patients who had made a good response to acute treatment could continue with blinded treatment for a further 24 weeks. In this extension phase, patients receiving 20 or 40 mg doses maintained their improvement, whereas those on the highest dose showed further improvements, compared to those continuing with placebo.

Two further studies provide conflicting evidence for the efficacy of higher doses of fluoxetine in long-term treatment [55, 58]. In a 2-year open-label study of patients who had responded to acute treatment (6 months), continuing with fluoxetine at a daily dose of 40 mg was found superior to stopping treatment, but no different to switching to 20 mg per day [57]. By contrast, a recent report [58] indicates that only a daily dose of 60 mg was significantly more efficacious than placebo in preventing relapse, among patients who had responded to acute treatment.

The relative efficacy of fluoxetine in OCD, compared to other treatments has also been evaluated [59, 60]. In a 10-week placebo-controlled study of fluoxetine and phenelzine involving 64 patients, fluoxetine (daily dose, 80 mg) was found superior to both placebo and phenelzine (daily dose, 60 mg) [59]. However, in another double-blind study of 55 patients receiving either fluoxetine (daily dose, 40 mg) or clomipramine (150 mg), there was no advantage for fluoxetine [60].

Fluoxetine has also been found efficacious in treating children and adolescents with OCD [55]. In a double-blind, placebo-controlled, fixed-dose (20 mg) crossover study in 14 children, aged between 8–15 years, treatment with fluoxetine was associated with a greater reduction (44%) in obsessive-compulsive psychopathology than was seen with placebo (27%).

Paroxetine

Three double-blind, placebo-controlled studies of paroxetine in the treatment of OCD have been published [61–63]. In the first study, 348 patients with OCD were allocated randomly to receive either placebo or fixed daily doses of paroxetine (20, 40 or 60 mg) for 12 weeks. The two higher doses were associated with significantly greater improvement than was seen with either placebo or the lowest dose of paroxetine, on both the Y-BOCS scale and the NIMH-OC scale [61].

In the second study [63], 406 patients with OCD received flexible daily doses of paroxetine (10–60 mg), clomipramine (25–250 mg) or placebo, again for 12 weeks. By the end of the study, paroxetine (mean daily dose at endpoint, 37.5 mg) was superior to placebo on all primary efficacy measures – the number of patients showing a reduction of at least 25% on the Y-BOCS, and the changes in Y-BOCS and NIMH-OC scores. Clomipramine (mean daily dose at endpoint, 113.1 mg) and paroxetine were similarly effective, but the overall tolerability of paroxetine was superior, with significantly fewer anticholinergic effects, and fewer adverse events leading to withdrawal.

The long-term efficacy of paroxetine in OCD is not yet established, although a preliminary report of a placebo-controlled relapse prevention study suggests that paroxetine has value in continuation therapy, after response to acute treatment [62].

Sertraline

Several double-blind, placebo-controlled studies have examined the efficacy of sertraline in the short-term and long-term treatment of OCD, both in adults and children. The first study [64] involved 87 patients with OCD, treated with flexible daily doses of sertraline (50–200 mg) for 8 weeks. Sertraline was found to be more efficacious than placebo across a range of outcome measures. A second flexible-dose study [65] which included 167 patients and lasted for 12 weeks, found similar results.

Sertraline has also been found efficacious in a fixed-dose study that included 324 patients with OCD [66]. Patients were randomly assigned to receive either placebo, or 50, 100 or 200 mg daily doses of sertraline. On all three main efficacy measures, sertraline was associated with significantly greater improvement than placebo, in the 50 mg and 200 mg groups. The patients who were treated with 100 mg per day did better than those receiving placebo on only one measure, which may reflect the rather high placebo response rates in this study. Those patients who responded to treatment could then continue treatment on a double-blind basis in a 1-year extension phase. In this study [67], there was an advantage for sertraline over placebo in the pooled analysis, patients showing further improvements over the year, but again the 100 mg daily dose group of patients fared less well than those patients receiving other doses of active treatment. The findings of this study are supported by a subsequent 2-year open-label extension study, in which prolonged treatment with sertraline was accompanied by further reductions in obsessive-compulsive psychopathology [68].

Sertraline has also been found efficacious in children and adolescents with OCD [69]. In a double-blind, placebo-controlled treatment study, 187 patients received either placebo or flexible daily doses of sertraline (50–200 mg) for 12 weeks. Patients treated with sertraline showed significantly greater improvements than those receiving placebo across a range of outcome measures, from the third week of the study. At the end-point, 42% of patients who received sertraline were much or very much improved, compared to 26% of patients allocated to placebo. The tolerability profile in children and adolescents was similar to that seen in adults. This study of sertraline supports the earlier finding that treatment with fluoxetine can be beneficial in some patients with childhood-onset OCD.

Sertraline appears to be at least as effective as clomipramine in the treatment of OCD. In a double-blind study, 168 patients received flexible doses of either sertraline (mean endpoint daily dose, 129 mg) or clomipramine (mean endpoint dose, 90 mg) for 16 weeks [70]. Sertraline was significantly more effective than clomipramine, probably because of the poor tolerability of clomipramine in this study, there being substantially more withdrawals due to side-effects with clomipramine (26%) than with sertraline (11%).

Citalopram

No placebo-controlled studies of citalopram in OCD were identified in this literature search. The best evidence for the efficacy of citalopram comes from a single-blind study of 30 patients, allocated randomly to receive either citalopram, fluvoxamine or paroxetine for 10 weeks, in which no difference was found between treatments [71]. Clearly, further studies need to be presented before citalopram can be considered an efficacious treatment in obsessive-compulsive disorder.

Synthesis

The SSRIs are clearly efficacious in patients with OCD, both in short-term and long-term treatment. An emerging literature supports the use of SSRIs in the treatment of children and adolescents with OCD, as well as in adults. OCD is usually a chronic disorder, waxing and waning in severity over time, and the magnitude of change during acute treatment studies can therefore be rather disappointing.

The relative efficacy and tolerability of clomipramine and the SSRIs in the management of patients with OCD has been discussed extensively. Although there are occasional studies indicating that an SSRI is more efficacious than clomipramine, four systematic reviews and meta-analyses have shown that treatment with clomipramine is marginally, but significantly more effective than treatment with SSRIs [72–75]. In turn, SSRIs are more effective than drugs which do not have serotonin re-uptake inhibition as part of their mechanism of action. The main advantage for SSRIs is their improved tolerability profile compared to clomipramine, which suggests that SSRIs should be considered a first-line pharmacological treatment for patients with OCD, clomipramine being reserved for those patients who do not show signs of improvement with fluvoxamine, fluoxetine, paroxetine or sertraline.

Social anxiety disorder (social phobia)

The treatment of patients with social phobia has received much attention in recent years, possibly because of increasing awareness of the burden imposed by this potentially lifelong condition. The effects of most of the SSRIs have been evaluated in short-term placebo-controlled randomised trials, there being as yet little information on the potential value of SSRIs in continuation treatment.

Fluvoxamine

The effects of fluvoxamine in social phobia have been investigated in two double-blind, placebo-controlled studies. In the first, single-centre, study [76] 30 patients were treated with placebo or a fixed daily dose of fluvoxamine (150 mg) for 12 weeks. A substantial improvement was seen in 7 (46%) of the 15 patients who were treated with fluvoxamine, but in only one patient (7%) who received placebo. There were significant advantages for fluvoxamine on measures of social and anticipatory anxiety, but no significant difference from placebo in phobic avoidance. In the second, multi-centre study [77] 92 patients received either placebo or flexible doses of fluvoxamine (mean daily dose at end-point, 202 mg) over 12 weeks. There were significant advantages for fluvoxamine on all social phobia rating scales from the eighth week of treatment, and at the end of the study there were significantly more responders with fluvoxamine treatment (42.9%) than with placebo (22.7%).

Fluoxetine

No placebo-controlled or comparator-controlled studies of fluoxetine in the treatment of social phobia have been published. There has been one investigation of fluoxetine in children with the syndrome of elective mutism, which may have some similarities to social phobia. In this double-blind, placebo-controlled study [78], children who had not responded to placebo treatment were randomly allocated to either continuing treatment with placebo or switched to fluoxetine, at a dose of 0.6 mg/kg/day. There were significant advantages for fluoxetine on parents' ratings of mutism and global change, but not on ratings made by teachers or health professionals. Most children remained substantially impaired at the end of the study.

Paroxetine

Three large double-blind, placebo-controlled, multi-centre studies have evaluated the effects of paroxetine in the short-term treatment of patients with social phobia [79, 80], (Data on file, SmithKline Beecham Pharmaceuticals). In the first study, conducted in North America, 187 patients were randomly allocated to receive either placebo or flexible daily doses (10–50 mg) of paroxetine for 12 weeks. At the end of the study, significantly more (55%) of the patients who were treated with paroxetine were rated as much or very much improved, compared to 23.9% of the patients who received placebo. There were also significant advantages for paroxetine over placebo in measures of social anxiety symptoms and phobic avoidance [79].

A second multi-centre study, conducted in Europe and South Africa [80] produced similar findings. A total of 290 patients were assigned randomly to receive either placebo or flexible doses of paroxetine (mean daily dose at endpoint, 34.7 mg) over 12 weeks of double-blind treatment. Significantly more patients who received paroxetine responded to treatment (65.7% *versus* 32.4%), and paroxetine was associated with significantly greater reductions in social anxiety symptoms and phobic avoidance, and with greater improvements in work, social and family life. A third placebo-controlled study, which employed fixed daily doses of paroxetine (20, 40 or 60 mg), found that there was little to be gained in increasing the dose of paroxetine above 40 mg per day, higher doses not being associated with greater improvement, but being linked to a greater side-effect burden (Data on file, SmithKline Beecham Pharmaceuticals).

There are at present no published large-scale studies of paroxetine in the long-term treatment of patients with social phobia, but an investigation of open-label acute treatment, followed by double-blind placebo-controlled discontinuation, found that continued treatment with paroxetine was efficacious in preventing relapse of illness [81].

Sertraline

Two placebo-controlled studies have examined the effects of sertraline in the acute treatment of patients with social phobia [82, 83]. In the first study, 12 patients underwent treatment with flexible daily doses of sertraline (50–200 mg) and placebo in a double-blind cross-over study. A statistically significant improvement in social anxiety symptoms was seen during treatment with sertraline, but not with placebo. This investigation is also noteworthy because participating patients preferred to be interviewed by a computer than by a clinician [82]. In the second placebo-controlled study, not yet reported in full, 233 patients again received flexible doses of sertraline or placebo over 12 weeks. At the end of the study, there were significant advantages for sertraline in measures of social anxiety symptoms and phobic avoidance, and in the proportion of patients who responded to treatment (sertraline, 52%; placebo 29%) [83].

Citalopram

There are as yet no published studies of the treatment of patients with social phobia with citalopram, but the efficacy of other SSRIs in this condition suggests that citalopram is likely to be efficacious.

Synthesis

A range of SSRIs have been found efficacious in the short-term treatment of patients with social phobia. Their potential efficacy in long-term treatment is not yet established, and their relative efficacy compared to other treatment approaches, including drug treatment with phenelzine and psychological treatment with cognitive behaviour therapy, is uncertain.

Generalised anxiety disorder

No placebo-controlled or comparator-controlled studies of treatment of patients with GAD with either fluvoxamine, fluoxetine, paroxetine, sertraline or citalopram have been published. The efficacy of SSRIs in mixed anxiety and depression, and in other chronic anxiety disorders suggests that SSRIs might have a role in the overall management of patients with GAD, but this has yet to be evaluated. The results of placebo-controlled studies with paroxetine are expected soon.

Post-traumatic stress disorder

There have been rather few placebo-controlled or comparator-controlled studies of SSRIs in the treatment of patients with post-traumatic stress disorder (PTSD). The results of placebo-controlled studies with paroxetine are expected shortly.

Fluoxetine

Two double-blind, placebo-controlled studies with fluoxetine have been performed. In the first study [84] 64 patients with PTSD were randomly allocated to receive placebo or fluoxetine, up to a maximum daily dose of 60 mg, for 5 weeks. The study sample comprised 31 combat veterans and 33 civilian patients. By the end of the study there were significant advantages for fluoxetine over placebo, in terms of overall PTSD psychopathology, this being particularly so in the civilian patients. Certain symptom clusters, such as hyperarousal and hostility, showed little change with fluoxetine treatment. A second placebo-controlled study of fluoxetine, exclusively in civilian patients, has been published [85]. A total of 53 patients received either flexible daily doses of fluoxetine (maximum dose, 60 mg) or placebo over 12 weeks. Treatment with fluoxetine was associated with significantly greater reductions in overall PTSD psychopathology, and with a greater likelihood of response (fluoxetine, 85%; placebo, 62%).

Sertraline

Two double-blind, placebo-controlled studies with sertraline have been performed [86, 87], though not yet published in full. Both studies employed a flexible-dose design, and lasted 12 weeks. In the first study [86], in which 208 patients received either placebo or sertraline (mean daily dose at end-point, 125 mg), there were advantages for sertraline in three measures of overall psychopathology, and no significant differences in the rate of discontinuation from treatment because of adverse experiences. In the second study [87], of 187 patients, there were significantly greater improvements with sertraline in three of four primary efficacy measures and all secondary measures, and again the rate of discontinuation because of side-effects was similar in the two groups.

Adjuvant treatment

Although SSRIs have been found efficacious in placebo-controlled and comparator-controlled treatment studies in groups of patients with differing anxiety disorders, many patients derive only minimal benefit from treatment, remaining substantially impaired by anxiety and depressive symptoms and phobic avoidance, with continuing impairment in social and occupational function. For these reasons, there is a clear need to establish the efficacy of adjuvant pharmacological treatments in the anxiety disorders, whereby an additional compound is combined with an SSRI, to which the patient has made only a minimal or partial response.

There have been few attempts to establish the efficacy of adjuvant treatments by using a double-blind, placebo-controlled design. Most of these approaches have been performed in patients with obsessive-compulsive disorder, refractory to treatment with clomipramine or SSRIs. All these studies have produced disappointing results. For example, the addition of buspirone was found unhelpful in the treatment of 14 patients who had made only a partial response to clomipramine [88]. Similarly discouraging findings were seen during buspirone augmentation of 13 patients who had responded poorly to earlier treatment with fluoxetine [89] or fluvoxamine [90].

In a series of studies, placebo-controlled lithium augmentation was found unhelpful in two groups of patients with OCD who had not responded to earlier treatment with fluvoxamine [91], whereas adjuvant haloperidol was found efficacious in a group of 34 patients particularly in those patients with co-morbid tics [92]. In further studies, desipramine was found ineffective in a group of 30 OCD patients who had shown little response to earlier treatment with fluoxetine, fluvoxamine or sertraline [93], and augmentation of fluvoxamine by pindolol was found ineffective in a group of 15 patients with OCD [94].

Conclusions

Although numerous double-blind placebo-controlled trials have shown that the SSRIs are efficacious in the short-term and long-term treatment of many patients suffering from a range of anxiety disorders, a substantial minority of patients show no response to treatment, and the magnitude of improvement in those that do respond is often disappointing. There is therefore an "efficacy gap" in the anxiety disorders, that could hopefully be filled by novel psychopharmacological approaches.

At present it is hard to predict which anxious patients will respond well to an SSRI, and who will respond only poorly, but a series of investigations suggest that greater severity and longer illness, an absence of previous remissions, the presence of psychiatric co-morbidity and certain physiological measures are associated with a poorer response to treatment [95–98]. This is an area that may be facilitated by the findings of pharmacogenomic investigations that are currently underway in patients with depressive disorders; if found helpful, it would be expected that the anxiety disorders would also come under scrutiny.

As a class, the SSRIs have a number of side-effects that many patients find unacceptable, including nausea, dizziness, initial insomnia and sexual dysfunction [99]. Many patients with anxiety disorders are exquisitely sensitive to the side-effects of psychotropic drugs, and as such there is also a "tolerability gap", which could be filled by the advent of new treatments with a more acceptable side-effect profile.

Finally, many patients have a preference for psychological approaches, fearing possible side-effects of drug treatment, or the risk of developing tolerance or dependence. There have been rather few well-designed controlled studies, where the effects of SSRIs are compared to psychological treatments – therefore a "knowledge gap" also exists, whereby clinicians cannot give a full picture of the relative strengths and weaknesses of differing approaches to the management of these often chronic and severe disorders.

Acknowledgements
This chapter is based upon a talk with the same title given at the annual meeting of the British Association for Psychopharmacology, held in Harrogate in July 1999. We are grateful to the editors for their advice regarding the development of the manuscript.

References

1 Anderson IM (1998) SSRIs versus tricyclic antidepressants in depressed inpatients: a meta-analysis of efficacy and tolerability. *Depression and Anxiety* 7 [suppl 1]: 11–17

2 Anderson IM, Tomenson BM (1999) Selective serotonin reuptake inhibitors versus tricyclic antidepressants: a meta-analysis of efficacy and tolerability. *J Affect Disord*; *in press*

3 Tollefson GD, Greist JH, Jefferson JW, Heiligenstein JH, Sayler ME, Tollefson SL, Koback K (1994) Is baseline agitation a relative contraindication for a selective serotonin reuptake inhibitor: a comparative trial of fluoxetine versus imipramine. *J Clin Psychopharmacol* 14: 385–391

4. Nutt DJ, George DT (1990) Serotonin and anxiety. *In*: GD Burrows, M Roth, R Noyes (eds): *Handbook of anxiety, Vol. 3, the neurobiology of anxiety*. Elsevier, Amsterdam, 189–221

5 Bell CJ, Nutt DJ (1998) Serotonin and panic. *Brit J Psychiat* 172: 465–471

6 Deakin JFW, Graeff FG (1991) 5-HT and mechanisms of defence. *J Psychopharmacol* 5: 305–315

7 Fineberg NA, Roberts A, Montgomery SA, Cowen PJ (1997) Brain 5-HT function in obsessive-compulsive disorder. Prolactin responses to d-fenfluramine. *Brit J Psychiat* 171: 280–282

8 Baldwin DS, Rudge SE (1995) The role of serotonin in depression and anxiety. *Int Clin Psychopharmacol* 9 (suppl. 4]: 41–45

9 Evans L, Kennardy J, Schneider P, Hoey H (1986) Effect of a selective serotonin uptake inhibitor in agoraphobia with panic attacks: a double blind comparison of zimelidine, imipramine and placebo. *Acta Psychiat Scand* 73: 49–53

10 Nilsson BS (1983) Adverse reactions in connection with zimelidine treatment: a review. *Acta Psychiat Scand* 308 (suppl): 115–119

11 den Boer JA, Westenberg HG, Kamerbeek WD, Verhoeven WM, Kahn RS (1987) Effect of serotonin uptake inhibitors in anxiety disorders; a double-blind comparison of clomipramine and fluvoxamine. *Int Clin Psychopharmacol* 2: 21–32

12 den Boer JA, Westenberg HG (1988) Effect of a serotonin and noradrenaline uptake inhibitor in panic disorder: a double-blind comparative study with fluvoxamine and maprotiline. *Int Clin Psychopharmacol* 3: 59–74

13 den Boer JA, Westenberg HG (1990) Serotonin function in panic disorder: a double blind placebo controlled study with fluvoxamine and ritanserin. *Psychopharmacology (Berlin)* 102: 85–94

14 Hoehn-Saric R, McLeod DR, Hipsley PA (1993) Effect of fluvoxamine on panic disorder. *J Clin Psychopharmacol* 13: 321–326

15 Woods S, Black D, Brown S et al. (1994) Fluvoxamine in the treatment of panic disorder in outpatients: a double-blind, placebo-controlled study. Presented at the Annual Meeting of the College of International Neuropsychopharmacology, Washington DC

16 Sandmann J, Lorch B, Bandelow B, Hartter S, Winter P, Hiemke C, Benkert O (1988)

Fluvoxamine or placebo in the treatment of panic disorder and relationship to blood concentrations of fluvoxamine. *Pharmacopsychiatry* 31: 117–121

17 Nair NP, Bakish D, Saxena B, Amin M, Schwartz G, West TE (1996) Comparison of fluvoxamine, imipramine, and placebo in the treatment of outpatients with panic disorder. *Anxiety* 2: 192–198

18 Bakish D, Hooper CL, Filteau MJ, Charbonneau Y, Fraser G, West DL, Thibaudeau C, Raine D (1996) A double-blind placebo-controlled trial comparing fluvoxamine and imipramine in the treatment of panic disorder with or without agoraphobia. *Psychopharmacol Bull* 32: 135–141

19 Van Vliet IM, Den Boer Westenberg HG, Slaap BR (1996) A double-blind comparative study of brofaromine and fluvoxamine in outpatients with panic disorder. *J Clin Psychopharmacol* 16: 299–306

20 Black DW Wesner R, Bowers W, Gael J (1993) A comparison of fluvoxamine, cognitive therapy, and placebo in the treatment of panic disorder. *Arch Gen Psychiat* 50: 44–50

21 Sharp DM, Power KG, Simpson RJ, Swanson V, Moodie E, Anstee JA, Ashford JJ (1997) Fluvoxamine, placebo and cognitive behaviour therapy used alone and in combination in the treatment of panic disorder and agoraphobia in primary care. *Brit J Gen Pract* 47: 150–155

22 Black DW, Wesner R, Bowers W, Monahan P, Gabel J (1995) Acute treatment response in outpatients with panic disorder: high versus low depressive symptoms. *Ann Clin Psychiat* 7: 181–188

23 Black DW, Monahan P, Wesner R, Gabel J, Bowers W (1996) The effect of fluvoxamine, cognitive therapy, and placebo on abnormal personality traits in 44 patients with panic disorder. *J Personality Disord* 10: 185–194

24 Sharp DM, Power KG, Simpson RJ, Swanson V, Anstee JA (1997) Global measures of outcome in a controlled comparison of pharmacological and psychological treatment of panic disorder and agoraphobia in primary care. *Brit J Gen Pract* 47: 150–155

25 Michelson D, Lydiard RB, Pollack MH, Tamura RN, Hoog SL, Tepner R, Demitrack MA, Tollefson GD, the Fluoxetine Panic Disorder Study Group (1998) Outcome assessment and clinical improvement in panic disorder: evidence from a randomized controlled trial of fluoxetine and placebo. *Amer J of Psychiat* 155: 1570–1577

26 Michelson D, Pollack M, Lydiard RB, Tamura R, Tepner R, Tollefson, the Fluoxetine Panic Disorder Study Group (1999) Continuing treatment of panic disorder after acute response: randomised, placebo-controlled trial with fluoxetine. *Brit J Psychiat* 174: 213–218

27 Bystritsky A, Rosen RM, Murphy KJ, Bohn P, Keys SA, Vapnik T. (1994–1995) Double-blind pilot trial of desipramine versus fluoxetine in panic patients. *Anxiety* 1: 287–290

28 Oehrberg S, Christiansen PE, Behnke E, Borup AL, Sverin B, Soegaard J, Callberg H, Judge R, Ohrstrom JK, Manniche PM (1995) Paroxetine in the treatment of panic disorder. A randomised double-blind, placebo-controlled study. *Brit J Psychiat* 167: 374–379

29 Ballenger JC, Wheadon DE, Steiner M, Bushnell W, Gergel IP (1998) Double-blind, fixed-dose, placebo-controlled study of paroxetine in the treatment of panic disorder. *Amer J of Psychiat* 155: 36–42

30 Lecrubier Y, Bakker A, Dunbar G, Judge R (1997) A comparison of paroxetine, clomipramine and placebo in the treatment of panic disorder. Collaborative Paroxetine Panic Study Investigators. *Acta Psychiat Scand* 95: 145–152

31 Lecrubier Y, Judge R (1997) Long-term evaluation of paroxetine, clomipramine and placebo in panic disorder. Collaborative Paroxetine Panic Study Investigators. *Acta Psychiat Scand* 95: 153–160

32 Burnham DB, Steiner MX, Gergle IP et al. (1995) Paroxetine long-term safety and efficacy in panic disorder and prevention of relapse: a double-blind study. Presented in poster session at the annual meeting of the American College of Neuropsychopharmacology, San Juan, Puerto Rico

33 Pohl RB, Wolkow RM, Clary CM (1998) Sertraline in the treatment of panic disorder: a double-blind multicenter trial. *Amer J of Psychiat* 155: 1189–1195

34 Pollack MH, Otto MW, Worthington JJ, Manfro GG, Wolkow R (1998) Sertraline in the treatment of panic disorder: a flexible-dose multicenter trial. *Arch Gen Psychiat* 55: 1010–1016

35 Londborg PD, Wolkow R, Smith WT, DuBoff E, England D, Ferguson J, Rosenthal M, Weise C (1998) Sertraline in the treatment of panic disorder. A multi-site, double-blind, placebo-controlled, fixed-dose investigation. *Brit J Psychiat* 173: 54–60

36 Wade AG, Lepola U, Koponen HJ, Pedersen V, Pedersen T (1997) The effect of citalopram in panic disorder. *Brit J Psychiat* 179: 549–553

37 Lepola UM, Wade AG, Leinonen EV, Koponen HJ, Frazer J, Sjodin I, Pettinen JTT, Pedersen T,

Lehto HJ (1998) A controlled, prospective, 1-year trial of citalopram in the treatment of panic disorder. *J Clin Psychiat* 59: 528–534

38 den Boer JA (1998) Pharmacotherapy of panic disorder: differential efficacy from a clinical viewpoint. *J Clin Psychiat* 59 (suppl 8]: 30–36

39 Boyer W (1995) Serotonin uptake inhibitors are superior to imipramine and alprazolam in alleviating panic attacks: a meta-analysis. *Int Clin Psychopharmacol* 10: 45–49

40 Baldwin DS, Birtwistle J (1998) The side-effect burden associated with drug treatment of panic disorder. *J Clin Psychiat* 59 (suppl 8]: 39–44

41 Mundo E, Bareggi SR, Pirola R, Bellodi L, Smeraldi E (1997) Long-term pharmacotherapy of obsessive-compulsive disorder: a double-blind controlled study. *J Clin Psychopharmacol* 17: 4–10

42 Perse TL, Greist JH, Jefferson JW, Rosenfeld R, Dar R (1987) Fluvoxamine treatment of obsessive-compulsive disorder. *Amer J of Psychiat* 144: 1543–1548

43 Goodman WK, Price LH, Rasmussen SA, Delgado PL, Heninger GR, Charney DS (1989) Efficacy of fluvoxamine in obsessive-compulsive disorder. A double-blind comparison with placebo. *Arch Gen Psychiat* 46: 36–44

44 Cottraux J, Mollard E, Bouvard M, Marks I, Sluys M, Nury AM, Douge R, Cialdella P (1990) A controlled study of fluvoxamine and exposure in obsessive-compulsive disorder. *Int Clin Psychopharmacol* 5: 17–30

45 Cottraux J, Mollard E, Bouvard M, Marks I (1993) Exposure therapy, fluvoxamine, or combination treatment in obsessive-compulsive disorder: one-year follow-up. *Psychiat Res* 49: 63–75

46 Greist JH, Jenike MA, Robinson DS, Rasmussen SA (1995) Efficacy of fluvoxamine in obsessive-compulsive disorder: results of a multicentre, double-blind, placebo-controlled trial. *Eur J Clin Res* 7: 195–204

47 Goodman WK, Kozak MJ, Liebowitz M, White KL (1996) Treatment of obsessive-compulsive disorder with fluvoxamine: a multicentre, double-blind, placebo-controlled trial. *Int Clin Psychopharmacol* 11: 21–29

48 Freeman CP, Trimble MR, Deakin JF, Stokes TM, Ashford JJ (1994) Fluvoxamine versus clomipramine in the treatment of obsessive compulsive disorder: a multicenter, randomized, double-blind, parallel group comparison. *J Clin Psychiat* 55: 301–305

49 Koran LM, McElroy SL, Davidson JR, Rasmussen SA, Hollander E, Jenike MA (1996) Fluvoxamine versus clomipramine for obsessive-compulsive disorder: a double-blind comparison. *J Clin Psychopharmacol* 16: 121–129

50 Milanfranchi A, Ravagli S, Lensi P, Marazziti D, Cassano GB (1997) A double-blind study of fluvoxamine and clomipramine in the treatment of obsessive-compulsive disorder. *Int Clin Psychopharmacol* 12: 131–136

51 Hohagen F, Winkelmann G, Rasche-Rule H, Hand I, Konig A, Munchau N, Hiss H, Geiger-Kabisch C, Kappler C, Schramm P et al (1998) Combination of behaviour therapy with fluvoxamine in comparison with behaviour therapy and placebo. Results of a multicentre study. *Brit J Psychiat* 35: 71–78

52 van Balkom AJLM, de Haan E, van Oppen P, Spinhoven P, Hoogduin KAL, van Dyck R (1998) Cognitive and behavioural therapies alone versus in combination with fluvoxamine in the treatment of obsessive compulsive disorder. *J Nerv Ment Dis* 186: 492–499

53 Montgomery SA, McIntyre A, Osterheider M, Sarteschi P, Zitterl W, Zohar J, Birkett M, Wood AJ (1993) A double-blind, placebo-controlled study of fluoxetine in patients with DSM-III-R obsessive-compulsive disorder. The Lilly European OCD Study Group. *Eur Neuropsychopharmacol* 3: 143–152

54 Tollefson GD, Rampey AH Jr, Potvin JH, Jenike MA, Rush AJ, Komiguez RA, Koran LM, Shear MK, Goodman WK, Genduso LA (1994) A multicenter investigation of fixed-dose fluoxetine in the treatment of obsessive-compulsive disorder. *Arch Gen Psychiat* 51: 559–567

55 Riddle MA, Scahill L, King RA, Hardin MT, Anderson GM, Ort SI, Smith JC, Leckman JF, Cohen DJ (1992) Double-blind, crossover trial of fluoxetine and placebo in children and adolescents with obsessive-compulsive disorder. *J Amer Acad Child Adolesc Psychiat* 31: 1062–1069

56 Tollefson GD, Birkett M, Koran L, Genduso L (1994) Continuation treatment of OCD: double-blind and open-label experience with fluoxetine. *J Clin Psychiat* 55 (suppl): 69–76

57 Ravizza L, Barzega G, Bellino S, Bogetto F, Maina G (1996) Drug treatment of obsessive-compulsive disorder (OCD): long-term trial with clomipramine and selective serotonin reuptake inhibitors (SSRIs). *Psychopharmacol. Bull.* 32: 167–173

58 Romano S, Goodman WK, Tamura R, Gonzalez J and Collaborative Research Group. Long-term treatment of obsessive compulsive disorder following acute response: a comparison of fluoxetine versus placebo; *submitted for publication*

59 Jenike MA, Baer L, Minichiello WE, Rauch SL, Buttolph ML (1997) Placebo-controlled trial of fluoxetine and phenelzine for obsessive-compulsive disorder. *Amer J of Psychiat* 154: 1261–1264

60 Lopez-Ibor JJ Jr, Saiz J, Cottraux J, Note I, Vinas R, Bourgeois M, Hernandez M, Gomez-Perez JC (1996) Double-blind comparison of fluoxetine versus clomipramine in the treatment of obsessive-compulsive disorder. *Eur Neuropsychopharmacol* 6: 111–118

61 Wheadon D, Bushnell WD, Steiner M (1993) A fixed dose comparison of 20, 40 or 60 mg of paroxetine in the treatment of obsessive-compulsive disorder. Presented at the American College of Neuropsychopharmacology Annual Meeting, Puerto Rico, December

62 Dunbar GC, Steiner M, Bushnell WD, Gergel I, Wheadon DE (1995) Long term treatment and prevention of obsessive compulsive disorder with paroxetine. *Eur Neuropsychopharmacol* 5: 372

63 Zohar J, Judge R (1996) Paroxetine versus clomipramine in the treatment of obsessive-compulsive disorder. OCD Paroxetine Study Investigators. *Brit J Psychiat* 169: 468–474

64 Chouinard G, Goodman WK, Greist J, Jenike M, Rasmussen S, White K (1990) Results of a double-blind placebo controlled trial of a new serotonin uptake inhibitor, sertraline, in the treatment of obsessive-compulsive disorder. *Psychopharmacol. Bull.*26: 279–284

65 Kronig MH, Apter J, Asnis G, Bystritsky A, Curtis G, Ferguson J, Landbloom R, Munjack D, Riesenberg R, Robinson D et al (1999) Placebo-controlled, multicenter study of sertraline treatment for obsessive-compulsive disorder. *J Clin Psychopharmacol* 19: 172–176

66 Greist JH, Chouinard G, DuBoff E, Halaris A, Kim SW, Koran L, Liebowitz M, Lydiard RB, Rasmussen S, White K et al (1995) Double-blind parallel comparison of three dosages of sertraline and placebo in outpatients with obsessive-compulsive disorder. *Arch Gen Psychiat* 52: 289–295

67 Greist JH, Jefferson JW, Kobak KA, Chouinard G, DuBoff E, Halaris A, Kim SW, Koran L, Liebowitz MR, Lydiard B et al (1995) A 1 year double-blind placebo-controlled fixed dose study of sertraline in the treatment of obsessive-compulsive disorder. *Int Clin Psychopharmacol* 10: 57–65

68 Rasmussen S, Hackett E, DuBoff E, Greist J, Halaris A, Koran LM (1997) A 2-year study of sertraline in the treatment of obsessive-compulsive disorder. *Int Clin Psychopharmacol* 12: 309–316

69 March JS, Biederman J, Wolkow R, Safferman A, Mardekian J, Cook EH, Cutler NR, Dominguez R, Ferguson J, Muller B et al (1998) Sertraline in children and adolescents with obsessive-compulsive disorder: a multicenter randomized controlled trial. *J Amer Med Assoc* 280: 1752–1756

70 Bisserbe JC, Lane RM, Flament MF (1997) A double-blind comparison of sertraline and clomipramine in outpatients with obsessive-compulsive disorder. *Eur Psychiat* 12: 82–93

71 Mundo E, Bianchi L, Bellodi L (1997) Efficacy of fluvoxamine, paroxetine, and citalopram in the treatment of obsessive-compulsive disorder: a single-blind study. *J Clin Psychopharmacol* 17: 267–271

72 Piccinelli M, Pini S, Bellantuono C, Wilkinson G (1995) Efficacy of drug treatment in obsessive-compulsive disorder. A meta-analytic review. *Brit J Psychiat* 166: 424–443

73 Greist JH, Jefferson JW, Kobak KA, Katzelnick DJ, Serlin RC (1995) Efficacy and tolerability of serotonin transport inhibitors in obsessive-compulsive disorder. *Arch Gen Psychiat* 52: 53–60

74 Stein DJ, Spadaccini E, Hollander E (1995) Meta-analysis of pharmacotherapy trials for obsessive-compulsive disorder. *Int Clin Psychopharmacol* 10: 11–18

75 Pigott TA, Seay SM (1999) A review of the efficacy of selective serotonin reuptake inhibitors in obsessive-compulsive disorder. *J Clin Psychiat* 60: 101–106

76 van Vliet IM, den Boer JA, Westenberg HG (1994) Psychopharmacological treatment of social phobia: a double blind placebo controlled study with fluvoxamine. *Psychopharmacology* (Berlin) 115: 128–134

77 Stein MB, Fyer AJ, Davidson JR, Pollack MH, Wiita B (1999) Fluvoxamine treatment of social phobia (social anxiety disorder): a double-blind, placebo-controlled study. *Amer J of Psychiat* 156: 756–760

78 Black B, Uhde TW (1994) Treatment of elective mutism with fluoxetine: a double-blind, placebo-controlled study. *J Amer Acad Child Adolesc Psychiat* 33: 701–703

79 Stein MB, Liebowitz Lydiard RB, Pitts CD, Bushnell W, Gergel I (1998) Paroxetine treatment of generalized social phobia (social anxiety disorder): a randomized controlled trial. *J Amer Med Assoc* 280: 708–713

80 Baldwin DS, Bobes J, Stein DJ, Scharwachter I, Faure M (1999) Paroxetine in social phobia/social anxiety disorder. Randomised, double-blind, placebo-controlled study. *Brit J Psychiat* 175: 120–126

81 Stein MB, Chartier MJ, Hazen AL, Kroft CD, Chale RA, Cote D, Walker JR (1996) Paroxetine in the treatment of generalized social phobia: open-label treatment and double-blind placebo-controlled discontinuation. *J Clin Psychopharmacol* 16: 218–222

82 Katzelnick DJ, Kobak KA, Greist JH, Jefferson W, Mantle JM, Serlin RC (1995) Sertraline for social phobia: a double-blind placebo-controlled crossover study. *Amer J of Psychiat* 152: 1368–1371

83 Van Ameringen M, Mancini C, Streiner D (1994) Sertraline in social phobia. *J Affect Disord* 31: 141–5

84 van der Kolk BA, Dreyfus D, Michaels M, Shera D, Berkowitz R, Fisler R, Saxe G (1994) Fluoxetine in posttraumatic stress disorder. *J Clin Psychiat* 55: 517–522

85 Connor KM, Sutherland SM, Tupler LA, Malik ML, Davidson JRT (1999) Fluoxetine in post-traumatic stress disorder. A randomised double-blind study. *Brit J Psychiat* 175: 17–22

86 Davidson J, van der Kolk Brady K, Rothbaum B, Sikes C, Farfel G (1997) Double-blind comparison of sertraline and placebo in patients with post-traumatic stress disorder. Presented at 10th ECNP, Vienna, Austria, September

87 Baker D, Brady K, Goldstein S, Farfel G (1998) Double-blind flexible-dose multicenter study of sertraline and placebo in outpatients with post-traumatic stress disorder. Presented at American College of Neuropsychopharmacology, Puerto Rico, December

88 Pigott TA, L'Heureux F, Hill JL, Bihari K, Berstein SE, Murphy DL (1992) A double-blind study of adjuvant buspirone hydrochloride in clomipramine-treated patients with obsessive-compulsive disorder. *J Clin Psychopharmacol* 12: 11–18

89 Grady TA, Pigott TA, L'Heureux F, Hill JL, Berstein SE, Murphy DL (1993) Double-blind study of adjuvant buspirone for fluoxetine-treated patients with obsessive-compulsive disorder. *Amer J of Psychiat* 150: 819–821

90 McDougle CJ, Goodman WK, Leckman JF, Holzer JC, Barr LC, McCance-Katz E, Heninger GR, Price LH (1993) Limited therapeutic effect of addition of buspirone in fluvoxamine-refractory obsessive-compulsive disorder. *Amer J of Psychiat* 150: 647–649

91 McDougle CJ, Price LH, Goodman WK, Charney DS, Heninger GR (1991) A controlled trial of lithium augmentation in fluvoxamine-refractory obsessive-compulsive disorder: lack of efficacy. *J Clin Psychopharmacol* 11: 175–184

92 McDougle CJ, Goodman WK, Leckman JF, Lee NC, Heninger GR, Price LH (1994) Haloperidol addition in fluvoxamine-refractory obsessive-compulsive disorder. A double-blind, placebo-controlled study in patients with and without tics. *Arch Gen Psychiat* 51: 302–308

93 Barr LC, Goodman WK, Anand A, McDougle CJ, Price LH (1997) Addition of desipramine to serotonin reuptake inhibitors in treatment-resistant obsessive-compulsive disorder. *Amer J of Psychiat* 154: 1293–1295

94 Mundo E, Gugliemo E, Bellodi L (1998) Effect of adjuvant pindolol on the antiobsessional response to fluvoxamine: a double-blind, placebo-controlled study. *Int Clin Psychopharmacol* 13: 219–224

95 Slaap BR, van Vliet IM, Westenberg HG, den Boer JA (1995) Phobic symptoms as predictors of nonresponse to drug therapy in panic disorder patients (a preliminary report). *J Affect Disord* 33: 31–38

96 Slaap BR, van Vliet IM, Westenberg HG, Den Boer JA (1996) Responders and non-responders to drug treatment in social phobia: differences at baseline and prediction of response. *J Affect Disord* 39: 13–19

97 Slaap BR, van Vliet IM, Westenberg HG, Den Boer JA (1996) MHPG and heart rate as correlates of nonresponse to drug therapy in panic disorder patients. A preliminary report. *Psychopharmacology* (Berlin) 127: 353–358

98 Thienemann M, Koran LM (1995) Do soft signs predict treatment outcome in obsessive-compulsive disorder? *J Neuropsychiat Clin Neurosci* 7: 218–222

99 Baldwin DS, Thomas SC, Birtwistle J (1997) Effects of antidepressant drugs on sexual function. *Int J Psychiat Clin Pract* 1: 47–58

Subtype-selective benzodiazepine receptor ligands

Guy Griebel, Ghislaine Perrault and David J. Sanger

Sanofi-Synthelabo, 31 avenue Paul Vaillant-Couturier, 92220 Bagneux, France

Introduction

Introduced over 30 years ago, benzodiazepines (BZs) quickly became the most widely used of all psychotropic drugs. Their marked anxiolytic, hypnotic, anti-convulsant and muscle relaxant properties and their relative safety, rapidly elevated BZs to the treatment of choice for common and recurrent conditions such as anxiety states, tension and insomnia. However, in recent years, attitudes toward these compounds have greatly changed, and growing awareness and concern about dependence liability, withdrawal phenomena and short- and long-term side-effects has brought the long-term use of these compounds into question [1, 2]. BZs produce their pharmacological effects by allosterically and positively modulating the action of GABA at $GABA_A$ receptors at specific sites which are referred to as BZ/ω receptors [3–5]. The search for compounds chemically unrelated to BZs with more specific therapeutic actions and without the concomitant unwanted effects has led to the development of drugs that selectively bind to specific BZ/ω receptor subtypes and/or show different efficacies at BZ/ω receptors. For example, studies in animals showed that the non-selective BZ/ω receptor partial agonists bretazenil, imidazenil, Ro 19-5663, Ro 19-5686 and Ro 41-3696 displayed comparable or even greater efficacy in anxiety models than BZs, but produced less motor impairment [6–11]. Furthermore, following repeated treatment with Ro 19-5663, Ro 19-5686, Ro 41-3696 and the selective $BZ/ω_1$ receptor agonist zolpidem in rodents, there was no evidence for tolerance and physical dependence as was observed with most BZs [12, 13]. This article gives an overview of the main pharmacological findings with subtype-selective BZ/ω receptor agonists. The focus is on a review of the results obtained in animal studies, but clinical findings are also considered.

Benzodiazepine-sensitive $GABA_A$ receptors

Based on the finding that all BZs displaced the binding of $[^3H]BZs$ in different brain regions in a monophasic manner, it was originally thought that there was a unique class of BZ receptors [14, 15]. However, the subsequent finding that compounds structurally unrelated to BZs such as the triazolopyridazine CL218872, the imidazopyridine zolpidem or certain β-carbolines such as abecarnil, display different affinity for BZ receptors in the cerebellum than those in the hippocampus or other brain regions, suggested the existence of two BZ-receptor subtypes [4, 5, 16]. These were named BZ_1 and BZ_2 [3, 4], also designated as ω_1 and ω_2, respectively [5]. Subsequent cloning from cDNA libraries which has identified nearly twenty related $GABA_A$ receptor subunits in mammals, indicated that the $GABA_A$ receptor encompasses a heterogeneous population of multiple subunits. $GABA_A$ receptors have a pentameric form and each receptor is assembled from a combination of subunits from seven different sequence families (α_{1-6}, β_{1-4}, γ_{1-3}, ρ_{1-3}, ε_1, π_1 and δ_1) [17–20]. Hence, a new classification of the $GABA_A$ receptor subtypes based on subunit structure was proposed [21]. As an illustration, the BZ/ω_1 subtype is now referred to as $GABA_{A1a}$ receptor since its pharmacology mimics that of the co-expressed recombinants $\alpha_1\beta_n,\gamma_2$ (Tab. 1). About 80% of all $GABA_A$ receptor subtypes contain the classical BZ/ω binding sites (for review, see [22]). The $GABA_{A1a}$ subtype is the most abundant, amounting to approximately 60% of the BZ/ω-sensitive $GABA_A$ receptors. It is expressed in numerous populations of GABAergic neurons, in particular in the cerebral cortex, basal forebrain, thalamus and cerebellum. The $GABA_{A2a}$, $GABA_{A3a}$ and $GABA_{A5a}$ subtypes are moderately abundant, each being associated with about 10% of $GABA_A$ receptors. They are most abundant in the olfactory bulbs and hippocampus (Tab. 1).

Table 1. Classification and distribution of the $GABA_A$ receptor subtypes containing the classical BZ/ω binding sites. Together, they represent about 80% of all $GABA_A$ recognition sites

$GABA_A$ receptor subtype	Subunit composition	Former classification	Regional preponderance
$GABA_{A1a}$	$\alpha_1\beta_n,\gamma_2$	BZ/ω_1	Cerebral cortex, thalamus, cerebellum, basal forebrain
$GABA_{A2a}$	$\alpha_2\beta_n,\gamma_2$	BZ/ω_2	Olfactory bulb, hippocampus, amygdala, striatum
$GABA_{A3a}$	$\alpha_3\beta_n,\gamma_2$	BZ/ω_2	Olfactory bulb, amygdala, septum, thalamus
$GABA_{A5a}$	$\alpha_5\beta_n,\gamma_2$	BZ/ω_2	Olfactory bulb, hippocampus, spinal trigeminal nucleus

Adapted from [21, 22]. n = 1–3.

Subtype-selective BZ/ω receptor ligands

A wide variety of ligands are now known to interact selectively with BZ/ω receptor subtypes, and the field is being researched with increased vigour in an effort to produce more selective agents. While there are BZ/ω receptor ligands

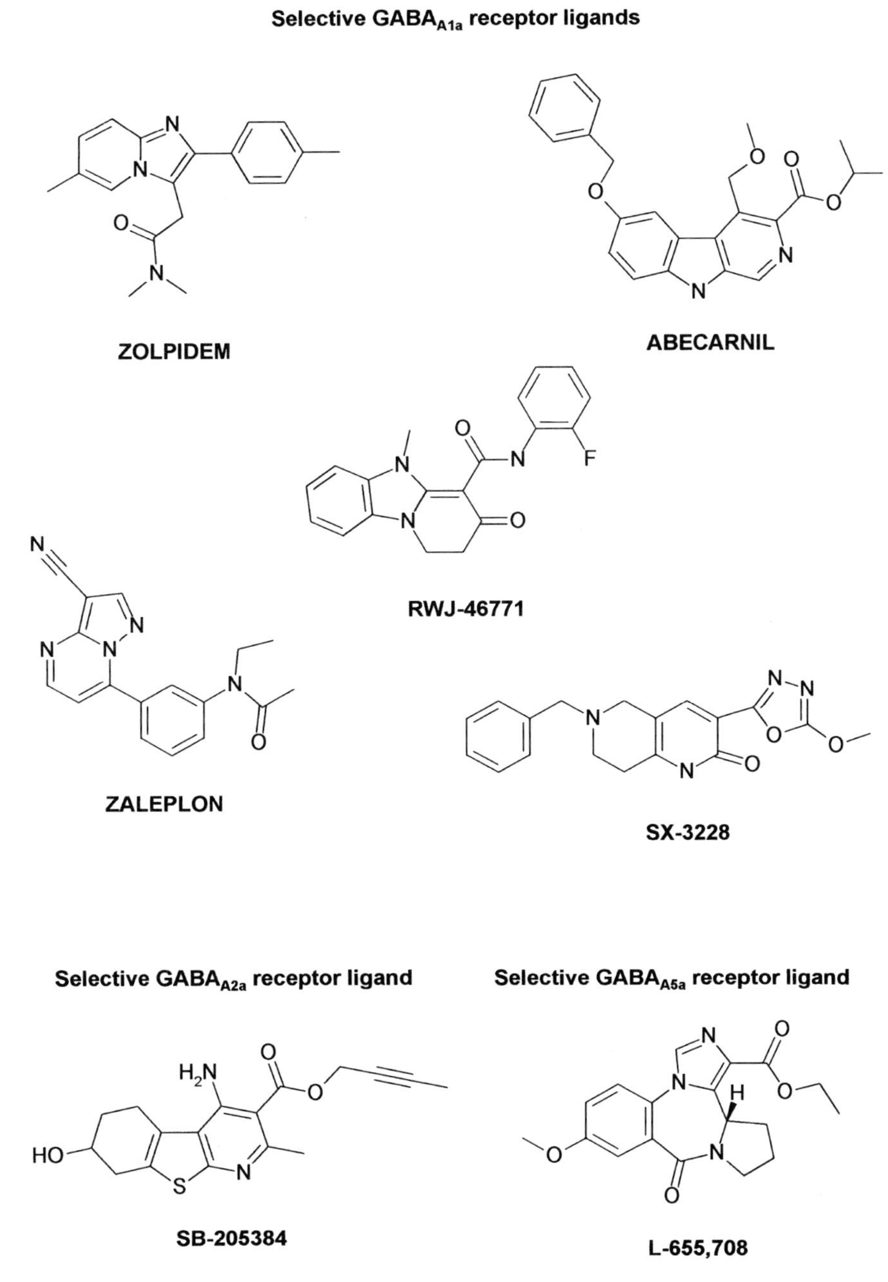

Selective GABA$_{A1a}$ receptor ligands

ZOLPIDEM

ABECARNIL

RWJ-46771

ZALEPLON

SX-3228

Selective GABA$_{A2a}$ receptor ligand   **Selective GABA$_{A5a}$ receptor ligand**

SB-205384

L-655,708

Figure 1. Examples of subtype-selective GABA$_A$ receptor ligands.

claimed in patents or shown to bind selectively for all BZ-sensitive GABA$_A$ receptor subtypes (Fig. 1), only compounds selective for the GABA$_{A1a}$ receptor subtype have been studied extensively. As illustrated in Figure 1, these latter include compounds with greatly varying chemical structures. The most widely studied $GABA_{A1a}$ receptor ligands are presented in Table 2. They include the imidazopyridine zolpidem, the β-carboline abecarnil, the pyrido[1,2-a]benzimidazole RWJ-46771, the pyrazolopyrimidine zaleplon and the 1,6-naphthyridin-2(1H)-one derivative SX-3228. While some of these compounds are marketed (zolpidem, zaleplon) or pre-registered (abecarnil), others have been discontinued during the preclinical phase (RWJ-46771 and SX-3228). This article gives an overview of the main experimental findings with zolpidem, abecarnil, RWJ-46771, zaleplon and SX-3228. Their pharmacological profiles were compared to that of the non-selective $GABA_A$ receptor full agonist diazepam.

Table 2. Effects of diazepam and several compounds described as selective for the $GABA_{A1a}$ receptor subtype on the binding of [³H] flumazenil to the native BZ/ω receptors in the rat cerebellum, a brain area enriched in $GABA_{A1a}$ receptors, and to the native BZ/ω receptors in the spinal cord, an area containing $GABA_{A2a}$, $GABA_{A3a}$ and $GABA_{A5a}$ sites

| | IC_{50} (nM) | | |
	Cerebellum	Spinal cord	$GABA_{A1a}$ receptor selectivity
Diazepam[1]	19	12	0.6
Zolpidem[2]	14	130	9.3
Abecarnil[1]	1.4	4	2.9
RWJ-46771[1]	0.4	1	2.5
Zaleplon[3]	78	570	7.3
SX-3228[1]	8.9	58	6.5

[1][24], [2][23], [3]Schoemaker, personal communication.

In vitro binding to BZ/ω receptor subtypes

Experiments on the inhibition of [³H] flumazenil binding to native BZ/ω receptor subtypes showed that zolpidem, abecarnil, RWJ 46771, zaleplon and SX-3228 were more potent in displacing [³H] flumazenil binding to membranes from rat cerebellum, a brain area enriched in $GABA_{A1a}$ receptors, than from spinal cord, an area containing $GABA_{A2a}$, $GABA_{A3a}$ and $GABA_{A5a}$ sites, thereby indicating selectivity for the $GABA_{A1a}$ receptor subtype ([23, 24], Schoemaker, personal communication). In contrast, the classical BZ diazepam displaced [³H] flumazenil binding in membranes from cerebellum and spinal cord non-selectively (Tab. 2). RWJ-46771 and abecarnil share similar high affinities (IC_{50}'s = 0.4 and 1.4 nM, respectively) for the $GABA_{A1a}$ receptor subtype. These values were slightly higher than those of SX-3228 and zolpidem, and considerably higher than that of zaleplon. Among the GABA$_{A1a}$ compounds, zolpidem, zaleplon and SX-3228 are the most selective, whereas RWJ-46771 and abecarnil are only moderately selective for the GABA$_{A1a}$ receptor subtype.

Intrinsic efficacy of selective GABA$_{A1a}$ receptor ligands

While differential binding affinity represents one form of selectivity for receptors, it may not be the only factor, because receptor subtype specific differences in modulatory efficacy may also be possible [25]. The intrinsic efficacy of BZ/ω receptor ligands can be assessed *in vitro* by studying the potentiation of Cl currents induced by rapid application of GABA in transfected cells expressing different combinations of GABA$_A$ receptors. Classical BZs, such as diazepam, interact with nearly all receptor subtypes with high efficacy. In contrast, partial agonists, typified by bretazenil or imidazenil act with reduced efficacy compared to diazepam at all receptors [25–27]. Among the selective GABA$_{A1a}$ receptor ligands, zolpidem showed a greater efficacy than diazepam in potentiating the GABA response in recombinant cells expressing the α_1 subunit, whereas it displayed a lower intrinsic activity than diazepam in transfected cells containing $\alpha_3\beta_2,\gamma_2$ subunits, and no activity at $\alpha_5\beta_2,\gamma_2$ combination [28] (Tab. 3). Abecarnil was reported to exert full agonistic effects on GABA$_A$ receptors containing the α_1 and α_3 subunits, whereas it behaved as a partial agonist at receptors containing the α_2 and α_5 subunits [29, 30]. The maximal potentiation achieved with zaleplon at α_1-, α_3- and α_5-containing combination was similar to that obtained by diazepam (Granger, personal communication). RWJ-46771 has been described as a partial agonist. However, in tissue preparations from rat cerebral cortex, it produced a GABA shift value (i.e. 1.6) somewhat greater than that observed with BZ/ω receptor partial agonists (i.e. 1.0) and close to that of the BZ/ω receptor full agonist lorazepam (i.e. 1.7) [31]. No data on the effects of SX-3228 on the potentiation of GABA response

Table 3. Efficacies of diazepam and several compounds described as selective for the GABA$_{A1a}$ receptor subtype in modulating GABA-induced chloride flux in recombinant systems expressing subtypes of GABA$_A$ receptors or in cortical tissues (RWJ-46771)

	Efficacy in modulating GABA-induced Cl flux
Diazepam	High at the at α_1-, α_3- and α_5-containing combinations[1]
Zolpidem	High at α_1-combination, low at α_3-combination, no efficacy at α_5-combination[1]
Abecarnil	High at α_1 and α_3-combinations, low at α_5-combination[2,3]
RWJ-46771	High in tissues from cerebral cortex[4]
Zaleplon	High at the at α_1-, α_3- and α_5-containing combinations[5]
SX-3228	?

[1][28] [2][29] [3][30] [4][31], [5]Granger, personal communication.

on transfected cells expressing different combinations of $GABA_A$ receptors have been published yet.

In vivo, the intrinsic efficacy of BZ/ω receptor ligands can be assessed by studying their ability to modify the latency to clonic seizures produced by isoniazid. Isoniazid inhibits glutamic acid decarboxylase, the enzyme that catalyses the synthesis of GABA from glutamic acid, thereby reducing the neuronal stores of GABA available for nerve impulse-mediated release of this transmitter [32]. The maximal delay in onset of isoniazid-induced seizures produced by a test compound may therefore be taken as an index of increased GABAergic function. It has been proposed as an *in vivo* measure of the intrinsic activity of BZ-ω receptor ligands at $GABA_A$ receptors [33]. Figure 2 shows that diazepam produced a larger increase in this measure than that seen with bretazenil, which is consistent with the well-acknowledged idea that diazepam shows higher intrinsic activity than bretazenil [24]. The selective $GABA_{A1a}$ receptor ligands showed different profiles in this test. Zolpidem and abecarnil produced a very large increase in the latency to clonic seizures produced by isoniazid, greater than those seen with diazepam and the other $GABA_{A1a}$ compounds [24, 34]. The efficacy of RWJ-46771 in increasing latency was slightly higher than that of diazepam and SX-3228, but considerably higher than that displayed by zaleplon [24]. Taken as a whole, these findings thus indicate that zolpidem and abecarnil may have greater intrinsic efficacy at $GABA_A$ receptors than RWJ-46771, diazepam, SX-3228 and zaleplon. It is noteworthy that

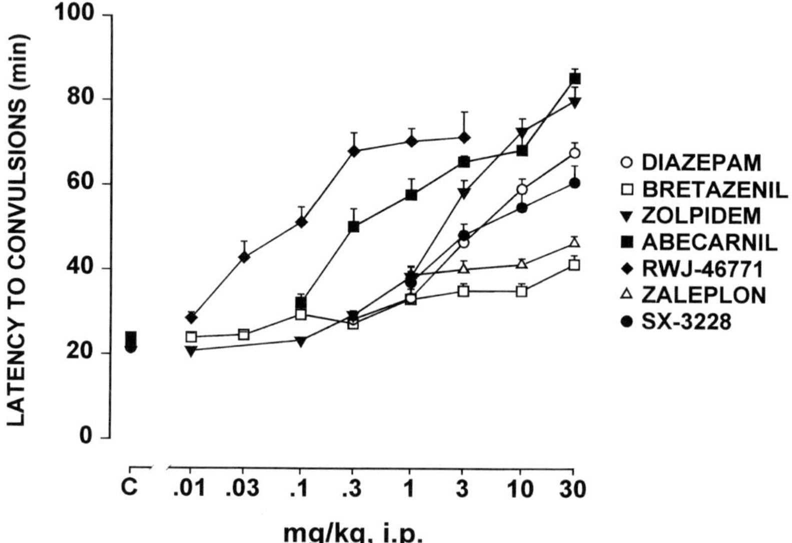

Figure 2. The anticonvulsant effects of diazepam, bretazenil and several selective $GABA_{A1a}$ receptor ligands against clonic seizures produced in mice by 800 mg/kg, s.c. of isoniazid. Data represent mean ± S.E.M. Adapted from [24, 34].

selective compounds with high efficacy in modulating GABA-induced chloride flux in recombinant systems also show high efficacy against isoniazid-induced convulsions, suggesting that this model is particularly sensitive to the action of selective $GABA_{A1a}$ receptor ligands.

Anxiolytic activity of selective $GABA_{A1a}$ receptor ligands

The anxiolytic-like properties of selective $GABA_{A1a}$ receptor ligands have been investigated in numerous studies. For example, abecarnil produced anxiolytic-like activities in several models in mice and rats, including the 4-plate test, the elevated plus-maze and the water-lick conflict test [35–38]. However, abecarnil was inactive in the free-exploration box, the light/dark test and in the defence test battery, three mouse models of anxiety [39, 40]. Table 4 summarises the effects obtained with zolpidem, abecarnil, RWJ-46771, zaleplon, SX-3228 and diazepam in five well-validated tests of anxiety under identical conditions. The tests include two conflict procedures (punished lever pressing and drinking tests in rats), two exploration models (elevated plus-maze in rats and light/dark test in mice) and a model based on defensive behaviours elicited in mice during confrontation with a natural threat (a rat) [24, 41].

Results showed that in the punished drinking test, all selective $GABA_{A1a}$ receptor ligands displayed anticonflict activity. In contrast, with the exception of SX-3228, selective compounds failed to modify punished responding in the lever pressing test. The anticonflict activity observed with the selective $GABA_{A1a}$ receptor ligands in the punished drinking test may have been contaminated by behavioural suppression as positive effects were observed at

Table 4. Minimal effective dose (MED) for anxiolytic-like activity and motor effects of diazepam and several selective $GABA_{A1a}$ receptor ligands

	MED (mg/kg, i.p.)				
	Rat			Mouse	
	Punished lever pressing	Punished drinking	Elevated plus-maze	Light/dark	Defence test Battery
Diazepam	2.5 (>5)	3	3 (>3)	4	1 (10)
Zolpidem	>3 (3)	3	1 (>1)	>3	10 (10)
Abecarnil	>1 (0.1)	3	0.3 (>3)	1	0.3 (0.3)
RWJ-46771	>0.3 (0.3)	1	>1 (1)	NT	0.03 (0.03)
Zaleplon	>3 (3)	1	0.3 (1)	10	3 (>10)
SX-3228	0.3 (1)	1	0.3 (0.3)	>0.3	0.03 (>1)

Motor effects (in brackets) were evaluated by measuring unpunished responding (Punished lever pressing), total arm entries (Elevated plus-maze) and line crossings (Defence test battery). NT: not tested. Adapted from [9, 11, 24, 39–41].

doses which impaired unpunished responding in the lever pressing procedure. One can assume that in the punished drinking test, motor deficits interfere less with responding than in the lever pressing model, so that anticonflict effects are still detectable. In the elevated plus-maze test, all drugs, except RWJ-46771, showed anxiolytic-like activity comparable to that of diazepam. Although the minimal effective dose for each compound was lower than that observed in the punished drinking test, anxiolytic-like activity appeared again at doses which were close to those producing impairment of motor activity as revealed by the data on the number of arm entries, a reliable measure of motor activity in this test. In the light/dark test, only abecarnil and zaleplon produced anxiolytic-like effects. However, it is important to note that the magnitude of the effects of zaleplon was small in comparison to diazepam. Moreover, in the case of abecarnil positive effects appeared at doses which also produced locomotor depression as indicated by results obtained in an actimeter which was run under identical test conditions. In the mouse defence test battery, only zaleplon and SX-3228 elicited anxiolytic-like activity at doses lower than those impairing motor activity. Moreover, like diazepam, zaleplon attenuated all defensive behaviours (e.g. flight, risk assessment, defensive threat and attack) recorded in this test battery.

Taken together, these data suggest that selective GABA$_{A1a}$ receptor ligands may have limited utility as anxiolytic agents and thus question the contribution of GABA$_{A1a}$ receptors in the anxiolytic activity of BZ ligands. A recent study using mice with point-mutated diazepam-insensitive GABA$_{A1a}$ receptors showed that they were still sensitive to the anxiolytic-like action of diazepam in the light/dark test, thereby indicating that different GABA$_A$ receptor subtypes may be involved in these effects [42]. However, the picture seems to be more complex. It was reported recently that the selective GABA$_{A1a}$ receptor antagonist β-CCT completely blocked the anxiolytic-like effects of diazepam in the light/dark test, suggesting that these effects were primarily mediated by GABA$_{A1a}$ receptors [43].

Alternatively, the lack of clear effects of the above-mentioned selective GABA$_{A1a}$ receptor ligands in anxiety models may be explained by the fact that their anxiolytic-like effects may have been confounded by decreases in locomotor activity. They all displayed high intrinsic efficacy as revealed by the findings from the isoniazid-induced convulsion test. Hence, it is possible that selective GABA$_{A1a}$ receptor ligands which behave as partial agonists at this receptor subtype may prove to produce fewer sedative effects, but retain anxiolytic properties. Clearly, further studies are needed before any definitive conclusion can be drawn on the contribution of selective GABA$_{A1a}$ receptor in the anxiolytic effects of BZ/ω receptor ligands and, therefore, on the anxiolytic potential of selective GABA$_{A1a}$ compounds.

The few clinical data available with abecarnil and zolpidem do not clarify the picture of the therapeutic potential of selective GABA$_{A1a}$ ligands as anxiolytics. One clinical study showed that zolpidem and the BZ triazolam displayed comparable efficacy in improving anxiety states of insomniac patients

[44]. In two dose-finding studies in subjects with generalised anxiety disorder (GAD), abecarnil demonstrated efficacy in global improvement ratings and on the Hamilton Anxiety Scale [45, 46]. Moreover, in a placebo-controlled study in patients with GAD, abecarnil was found as efficacious as the BZ alprazolam [47]. However, it is worth mentioning that the higher doses of abecarnil had a high incidence of CNS sedative adverse effects.

Central depressant effects of selective $GABA_{A1a}$ receptor ligands

Central depressant effects of traditional BZs generally seen as sedation, ataxia or myorelaxation are usually manifested at doses higher than those producing anxiolytic-like actions. For example, Figure 3 shows that diazepam impaired the performance of rats in the actimeter, the rotarod and the loaded grid tests (three models generally used to examine the sedative, ataxic and myorelaxant properties of psychoactive drugs, respectively) within a dose-range (3–10 mg/kg) which was slightly higher than that producing anxiolytic-like activity (2.5–3 mg/kg) (Tab. 4) [24]. Following the initial finding that the selective $GABA_{A1a}$ receptor ligand CL218,872 produced a motor deficit on an inclined plane in rats at doses much higher than those increasing punished responding in the Vogel conflict test [48], it was suggested that drugs with selectivity for $GABA_{A1a}$ receptors may have less propensity to produce ataxia and muscle relaxation than non-selective compounds. This idea was strengthened by results from several studies showing that the selective $GABA_{A1a}$ receptor ligands zolpidem, abecarnil and alpidem induced muscle relaxation and ataxia at doses much higher than those producing other pharmacological effects [49–52]. As illustrated by Figure 3, the overall profile of central-depressant effects of the selective $GABA_{A1a}$ compounds is quite different from that displayed by the non-selective BZ/ω receptor agonist diazepam. Unlike diazepam, which significantly impaired motor performance in the actimeter, rotarod and loaded grid tests at the same doses, zolpidem, abecarnil, RWJ 46771 and SX-3228 induced myorelaxation at doses which were 3 to 10 times higher than those needed to decrease exploratory activity. Overall, these findings suggest that the $GABA_{A1a}$ subtype is not primarily involved in mediating the myorelaxant effects of BZ/ω receptor agonists. Consonant with this view is a recent finding which showed that the selective receptor antagonist β-CCT did not block the myorelaxant effects of diazepam [43]. Moreover, it was reported that mice lacking a diazepam-sensitive α_1 subunit still displayed muscle relaxation following the administration of diazepam [42]. As yet it is unclear which $GABA_A$ receptor subtype mediates the myorelaxant effects of BZ/ω receptor agonists. Nevertheless, the fact that the relative proportion of $GABA_{A3a}$ and $GABA_{A5a}$ sites are particularly high in the spinal cord [22] might indicate that these receptors play a particularly important role in these effects.

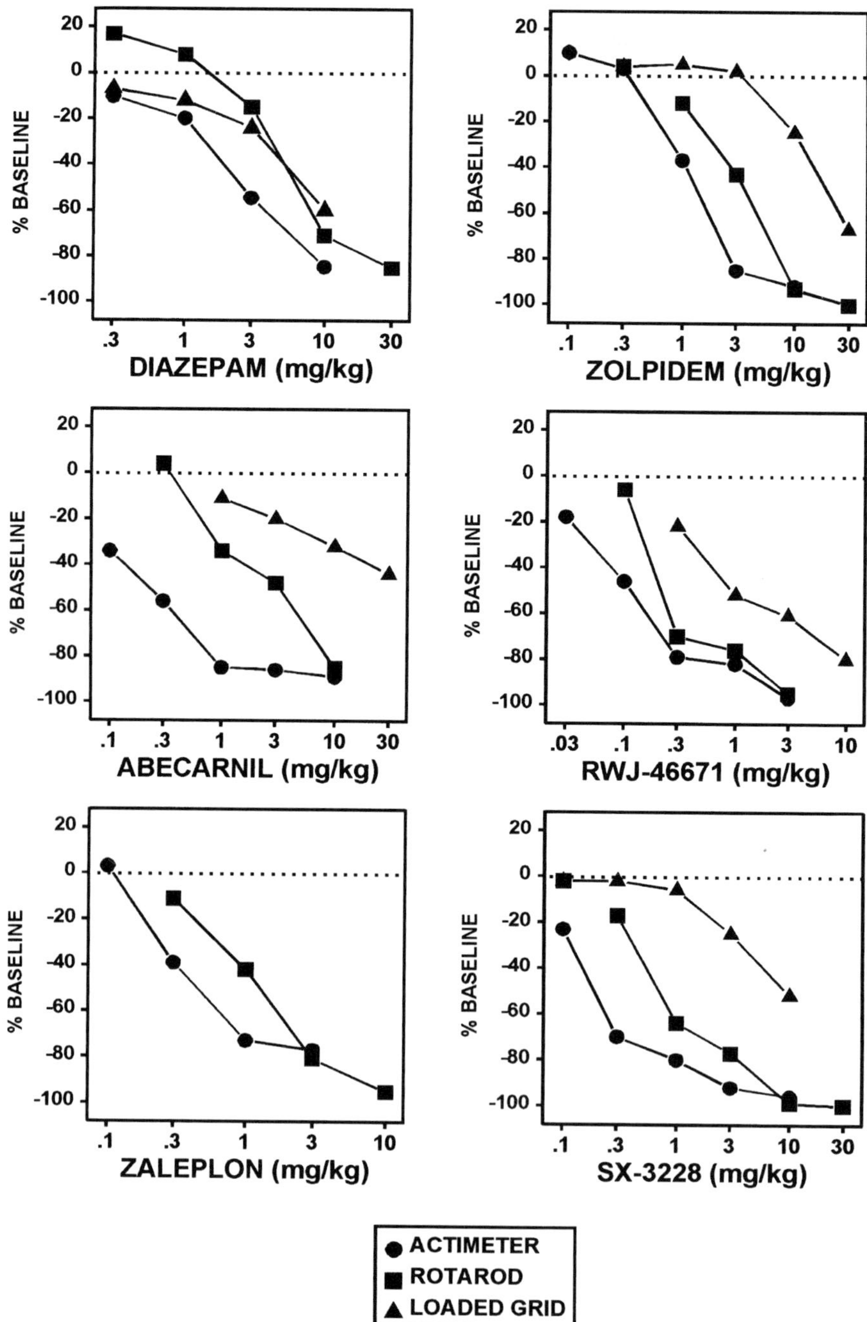

Figure 3. Effects of diazepam and several selective GABA$_{A1a}$ receptor ligands on tests measuring spontaneous locomotor activity (actimeter), ataxia (rotarod) and myorelaxation (loaded grid) in rats. Data are expressed as percentage of baseline levels. Adapted from [24].

Cognitive effects of selective GABA$_{A1a}$ receptor ligands

Anterograde amnesia is one of the troublesome adverse effects of the BZs, especially when they are used as tranquillisers. In animal procedures, BZs can give rise to actions indicating disturbances in learning [53]. Passive avoidance tests have been extensively used for studying the effects of BZs on learning and memory. These studies showed that administration of a BZ before the first trial produces a response deficit on the second trial, indicating a failure of acquisition. The selective GABA$_{A1a}$ receptor ligands zolpidem and alpidem have also been studied in passive avoidance tests in mice [13, 54]. Results showed that although both compounds disrupted the acquisition of conditioned fear, these effects occurred only at doses which greatly decreased locomotor activity, suggesting that a learning deficit may have been secondary to an action on motor performance. In contrast, diazepam disrupted learning at doses lower than those impairing motor activity. A comparative study of the effects of abecarnil and diazepam in a three-panel runway task has shown that the former drug impaired only working memory, whereas diazepam markedly impaired both reference and working memory. Moreover, the effects of abecarnil on working memory disappeared rapidly within 2 to 3 days of repeated treatment, whereas that of diazepam persisted during 14 days of repeated treatment [55].

Several clinical studies have described the effects of selective GABA$_{A1a}$ receptor ligands on various tests of memory. Zolpidem and alpidem have been found to produce impairments in a number of tests of recognition and recall, but these effects occurred at doses normally used for sleep-induction (zolpidem) or at doses higher than those recommended for the treatment of anxiety (alpidem) (for review, see [56]). In a study involving a comparison between abecarnil and lorazepam, Hege and colleagues [57] showed that these drugs impaired performance of healthy volunteers in tests of cognitive functions including memory encoding. However, abecarnil produced substantially less impairment than lorazepam. In another study, zaleplon and lorazepam were found to display similar impairment profiles in tests of cognitive functions, but recovery was rapid with zaleplon, whereas impairment induced by lorazepam persisted throughout the post-drug testing sessions [58]. In addition, zaleplon administered up to six times the dose normally used to induce sleep (ie 60 mg) did not affect the performance of healthy volunteers in a word recall test [59].

Taken together, both animal and clinical studies indicate that although selective GABA$_{A1a}$ receptor ligands may interfere with learning and memory processes, these effects usually occur at high and sedative doses.

Discriminative stimulus effects of selective GABA$_{A1a}$ receptor ligands

With BZ/ω receptor ligands, drug discrimination procedures provide additional information that assists in identifying receptor mechanisms involved in the actions of these drugs. The stimulus effects of BZs has been analysed in great detail following early studies using chlordiazepoxide [60] and diazepam [61]. In general, there is complete cross substitution between different BZs. Figure 4 shows the effects of several selective GABA$_{A1a}$ receptor ligands in rats trained to discriminate chlordiazepoxide [62]. In contrast to results obtained with non-

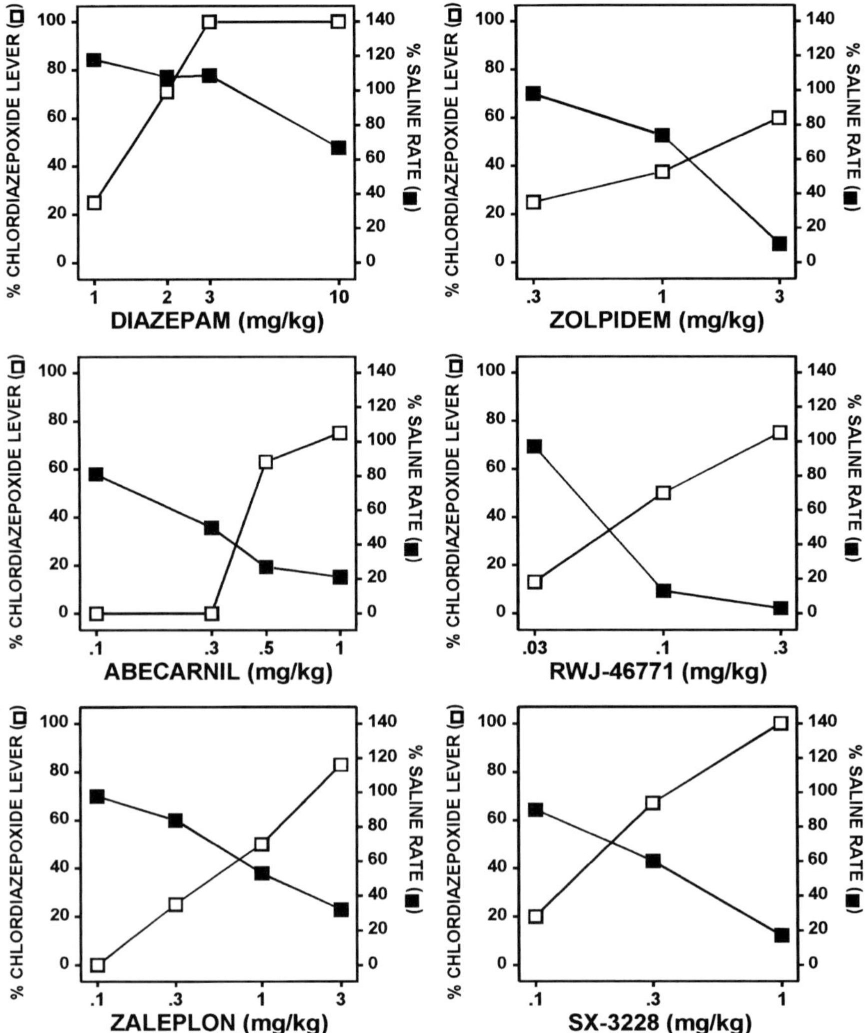

Figure 4. Effects of diazepam and several selective GABA$_{A1a}$ receptor ligands in rats trained to discriminate chlordiazepoxide (5 mg/kg) from saline. The results are shown as the percentage of animals responding on the chlordiazepoxide lever and the average response rate expressed as the percentage of response rates after saline injection. Adapted from [62].

selective compounds, these selective agents produced only partial substitution for the chlordiazepoxide cue and this activity was apparent only at sedative doses. These results show that this stimulus is mediated by $GABA_A$ receptor subtypes other than $GABA_{A1a}$. In line with this hypothesis, it has been demonstrated that there is a strong and significant correlation between drug lever responding following the administration of a variety of selective and non-selective BZ/ω receptor ligands, and *in vivo* displacement of [^{3}H]-flumazenil in the spinal cord, a region enriched in $GABA_{A5a}$ receptors (r = 0.96) [63]. The use of $GABA_{A5a}$ selective agents would provide more direct evidence that this receptor subtype is of relatively greater importance than the $GABA_{A1a}$ receptor in mediating the discriminative stimulus produced by chlordiazepoxide. Other experiments have used the $GABA_{A1a}$ selective agents zolpidem, alpidem, CL218,872 and zaleplon as training drugs in drug discrimination experiments with rats [62]. The results of these experiments showed differences between the effects of these compounds and non-selective agents suggesting that the discriminative cues may have been mediated by activity at the $GABA_{A1a}$ receptor subtype.

Effects of selective $GABA_{A1a}$ receptor ligands following repeated administration

Long-term administration of BZs is often associated with the development of tolerance. Drug tolerance has been defined as the process by which the effects of the same dose of a drug decrease with repeated administration. These effects are particularly well established for anticonvulsant and central depressant activities, but are not observed frequently in tests that assess anxiolytic-like activity [64]. Studies with the selective $GABA_{A1a}$ receptor ligands zolpidem, alpidem and zaleplon showed that these drugs did not give rise to tolerance to their anticonvulsant effects against isoniazid-, pentylenetetrazole- and/or bicuculline-induced convulsions in mice following repeated administration, while marked tolerance was observed with the BZs midazolam and diazepam [12, 34, 65]. Similarly, little tolerance was observed to the decrease in rates of operant responding produced in rats by zolpidem and CL 218,872, whereas clear tolerance was found with chlordiazepoxide, midazolam and triazolam [66–68]. Although in one study abecarnil was also found to produce little tolerance to its anticonvulsant effects against pentylenetetrazole-induced seizures following repeated administration for 10 days [55], in another study the drug was reported to lose anticonvulsant activity after 4 weeks of treatment [69]. The authors of the latter study discussed several possible reasons which may account for this discrepancy such as the use of an inadequate study design for obtaining predictable information on the tolerance of BZ/ω receptor ligands. Despite these latter findings, there is a great deal of evidence that chronic treatment with selective $GABA_{A1a}$ receptor ligands produces little or no tolerance to their anticonvulsant activity.

Numerous studies have documented withdrawal syndromes following abrupt discontinuation of long-term BZ treatment [64]. During withdrawal, the original anxiety symptoms often return in a more intense form. This phenomenon has also been described in laboratory research [56]. In animals, BZ-induced withdrawal signs can be quantified with a variety of behavioural and physiological measures and range from convulsions to subtle behavioural changes indicative of increased anxiety. Perrault et al. [12, 65] used increased sensitivity to convulsant drugs as a measure of physiological dependence to show that repeated treatment with the selective $GABA_{A1a}$ receptor ligands zolpidem and alpidem for 10 days did not modify sensitivity to convulsions induced by isoniazid, pentylenetetrazole or β-CCM. By contrast, in these studies, diazepam and midazolam produced increased sensitivity to all convulsant challenges. A similar lack of increased sensitivity to seizures induced by electroshock was observed following chronic zolpidem and CL218,872 [70]. Several studies with abecarnil have also found little or no evidence that repeated administration with this drug induces BZ-like dependence [71–74]. For example, Steppuhn and colleagues showed that mice withdrawn from repeated administration of abecarnil for 12 days displayed no anxiety and no changes in seizure susceptibility and muscle tone, unlike those treated chronically with diazepam which showed increased anxiety, muscle rigidity and seizures. In another study, chronic administration of abecarnil in baboons produced only transient signs of a mild withdrawal syndrome after drug discontinuation [72].

Clinical studies with zolpidem [75–79], alpidem [80] and zaleplon [81] have also indicated that a withdrawal syndrome does not occur with these drugs under conditions where such a syndrome is observed with some BZs. Although in two clinical trials with abecarnil there was no evidence for signs of withdrawal after drug discontinuation [47, 82], in another study, withdrawal symptoms emerged in patients who abruptly discontinued abecarnil (particularly at the higher dosage) but only in those receiving a longer duration of treatment [83].

Taken as a whole, these results with zolpidem, alpidem, abecarnil and zaleplon suggest that selective $GABA_{A1a}$ receptor ligands may give rise to little or no physiological dependence.

Final comment

It is clear from the above data that compounds which display selectivity for the $GABA_{A1a}$ receptor subtype offer several clinical advantages over traditional BZs. So far only compounds with high intrinsic efficacy at the $GABA_{A1a}$ receptor subtype have been described. Because of their high propensity to produce sedation, these compounds are useful in the clinical management of sleep disorders, but their utility in the treatment of anxiety disorders is limited. Selective compounds with partial agonistic activity at the $GABA_{A1a}$ receptor subtype may circumvent the problem of sedation and may thus represent a valid alternative to agents currently used for the treatment of anxiety disorders.

References

1 Lader M (1994) Benzodiazepines: a risk-benefit profile. *CNS Drugs* 1: 377–387
2 Woods JH, Winger G (1995) Current benzodiazepine issues. *Psychopharmacology* 118: 107–115
3 Squires RF, Benson DI, Braestrup C, Coupet J, Klepner CA, Myers V, Beer B (1979) Some properties of brain specific benzodiazepine receptors: new evidence for multiple receptors. *Pharmacol Biochem Behav* 10: 825–830
4 Sieghart W, Schuster A (1984) Affinity of various ligands for benzodiazepine receptors in rat cerebellum and hippocampus. *Pharmacol Biochem Behav* 33: 4033–4038
5 Langer SZ, Arbilla S (1988) Imidazopyridines as a tool for the characterization of benzodiazepine receptors: a proposal for a pharmacological classification as ω receptor subtypes. *Pharmacol Biochem Behav* 29: 763–766
6 Martin JR, Pieri L, Bonetti EP, Schaffner R, Burkard WP, Cumin R, Haefely WE (1988) Ro 16-6028: a novel anxiolytic acting as a partial agonist at the benzodiazepine receptor. *Pharmacopsychiatry* 21: 360–362
7 Giusti P, Ducic I, Puia G, Arban R, Walser A, Guidotti A, Costa E (1993) Imidazenil: a new partial positive allosteric modulator of gamma-aminobutyric acid (GABA) action at GABA$_A$ receptors. *J Pharmacol Exp Ther* 266: 1018–1028
8 Martin JR, Moreau JL, Jenck F (1995) Evaluation of the dependence liability of quinolizinones acting as partial agonists at the benzodiazepine receptor. *Drug Develop Res* 36: 141–149
9 Sanger DJ (1995) The behavioural effects of novel benzodiazepine (ω) receptor agonists and partial agonists: Increases in punished responding and antagonism of the pentylenetetrazole cue. *Behav Pharmacol* 6: 116–126
10 Sanger DJ, Joly D, Perrault G (1995) Benzodiazepine (ω) receptor partial agonists and the acquisition of conditioned fear in mice. *Psychopharmacology* 121: 104–108
11 Griebel G, Sanger DJ, Perrault G (1996) The use of the rat elevated plus-maze to discriminate between non-selective and BZ-1 (ω1) selective, benzodiazepine receptor ligands. *Psychopharmacology* 124: 245–254
12 Perrault G, Morel E, Sanger DJ, Zivkovic B (1992) Lack of tolerance and physical dependence upon repeated treatment with the novel hypnotic zolpidem. *J Pharmacol Exp Ther* 263: 298–303
13 Zivkovic B, Perrault G, Sanger D (1992) Receptor subtype-selective drugs: a new generation of anxiolytics and hypnotics. *In*: J Mendlewitz, G Racagni (eds): *Target receptors for anxiolytics and hypnotics: from molecular pharmacology to therapeutics.* Karger, Basel, 55–73
14 Braestrup C, Squires RF (1977) Specific benzodiazepine receptors in rat brain characterized by high-affinity (^{3}H)diazepam binding. *Proc Natl Acad Sci USA* 74: 3805–3809
15 Mohler H, Okada T (1977) Benzodiazepine receptor: demonstration in the central nervous system. *Science* 198: 849–851
16 Lippa AS, Beer B, Sano MC, Vogel RA, Meyerson LR (1981) Differential ontogeny of type 1 and type 2 benzodiazepine receptors. *Life Sci* 28: 2343–2347
17 Burt DR, Kamatchi GL (1991) GABA$_A$ receptor subtypes: from pharmacology to molecular biology. *Faseb* 5: 2916–2923
18 Davies PA, Hanna MC, Hales TG, Kirkness EF (1997) Insensitivity to anaesthetic agents conferred by a class of GABA$_A$ receptor subunit. *Nature* 385: 820–823
19 Hedblom E, Kirkness EF (1997) A novel class of GABA$_A$ receptor subunit in tissues of the reproductive system. *J Biol Chem* 272: 15346–15350
20 Whiting PJ, McAllister G, Vassilatis D, Bonnert TP, Heavens RP, Smith DW, Hewson L, ODonnell R, Rigby MR, Sirinathsinghji DJ et al (1997) Neuronally restricted RNA splicing regulates the expression of a novel GABAA receptor subunit conferring atypical functional properties. *J Neurosci* 17: 5027–5037
21 Barnard EA, Skolnick P, Olsen RW, Mohler H, Sieghart W, Biggio G, Braestrup C, Bateson AN, Langer SZ (1998) International Union of Pharmacology. XV. Subtypes of γ-aminobutyric acid$_A$ receptors: Classification on the basis of subunit structure and receptor function. *Pharmacol Rev*

50: 291–313

22 Fritschy JM, Mohler H (1995) GABA$_A$-receptor heterogeneity in the adult rat brain: Differential regional and cellular distribution of seven major subunits. *J Comp Neurol* 359: 154–194

23 Benavides J, Peny B, Durand A, Arbilla S, Scatton B (1992) Comparative *in vivo* and *in vitro* regional selectivity of central ω (benzodiazepine) site ligands in inhibiting [^{3}H] flumazenil binding in the rat central nervous system. *J Pharmacol Exp Ther* 263: 884–896

24 Griebel G, Perrault G, Tan S, Schoemaker H, Sanger DJ (1999) Comparison of the pharmacological properties of classical and novel BZ-ω receptor ligands. *Behav Pharmacol* 10: 483–495

25 *Puia G, Ducic I, Vicini S, Costa E* (1992) Molecular mechanisms of the partial allosteric modulatory effects of bretazenil at gamma-aminobutyric acid type A receptor. *Proc Natl Acad Sci USA* 89: 3620–3624

26 Haefely W, Martin JR, Schoch P (1990) Novel anxiolytics that acts as partial agonists at benzodiazepine receptors. *Trends Pharmacol Sci* 11: 452–456

27 Wafford KA, Whiting PJ, Kemp JA (1993) Differences in affinity and efficacy of benzodiazepine receptor ligands at recombinant γ-aminobutyric acid receptor subtypes. *Mol Pharmacol* 43: 240–244

28 Depoortere H, Granger P, Biton B, Avenet P, Faure C, Graham D, Langer SZ, Scatton B (1994) Functional and pharmacological properties of $\alpha_1\beta_2\gamma_2$, $\alpha_3\beta_2\gamma_2$ and $\alpha_5\beta_2\gamma_2$ subtypes of GABA$_A$ receptors transiently expressed in HEK 293 cells. *Can J Physiol Pharmacol* 72 (suppl. 1): 338

29 Knoflach F, Drechsler U, Scheurer L, Malherbe P, Mohler H (1993) Full and partial agonism displayed by benzodiazepine receptor ligands at recombinant γ-aminobutyric acid$_A$ receptor. *J Pharmacol Exp Ther* 266: 385–391

30 Pribilla I, Neuhaus R, Huba R, Hillmann M, Turner JD, Stephens DN, Schneider HH (1993) Abecarnil is a full agonist at some, and a partial agonist at other recombinant GABA$_A$ receptor subtypes. *In*: DN Stephens (ed.): *Anxiolytic β-carbolines*. Springer-Verlag, Berlin, 50–61

31 Maryanoff BE, Ho W, McComsey DF, Reitz AB, Grous PP, Nortey SO, Shank RP, Dubinsky B, Taylor RJ, Gardocki JF (1995) Potential anxiolytic agents. Pyrido[1,2-alpha]benzimidazoles: A new structural class of ligands for the benzodiazepine binding site on GABA-A receptors. *J Med Chem* 38: 16–20

32 Löscher W, Frey HH (1977) Effect of convulsant and anticonvulsant agents on level and metabolism of gamma-aminobutyric acid in mouse brain. *Naunyn-Schmied Arch Pharmacol* 296: 263–269

33 Mao CC, Guidotti A, Costa E (1975) Evidence for an involvement of GABA in the mediation of the cerebellar cGMP decrease and the anticonvulsant action diazepam. *Naunyn-Schmied Arch Pharmacol* 289: 369–378

34 Sanger DJ, Morel E, Perrault G (1996) Comparison of the pharmacological profiles of the hypnotic drugs, zaleplon and zolpidem. *Eur J Pharmacol* 313: 35–42

35 Stephens DN, Schneider HH, Kehr W, Andrews JS, Rettig KJ, Turski L, Schmiechen R, Turner JD, Jensen LH, Petersen EN (1990) Abecarnil, a metabolically stable, anxioselective beta-carboline acting at benzodiazepine receptors. *J Pharmacol Exp Ther* 253: 334–343

36 Sanger DJ, Perrault G, Morel E, Joly D, Zivkovic B (1991) Animal models of anxiety and the development of novel anxiolytic drugs. *Prog Neuro-Psych Biol Psychiat* 15: 205–212

37 Jones GH, Schneider C, Schneider HH, Seidler J, Cole BJ, Stephens DN (1994) Comparison of several benzodiazepine receptor ligands in two models of anxiolytic activity in the mouse: An analysis based on fractional receptor occupancies. *Psychopharmacology* 114: 191–199

38 Stephens DN, Voet B (1994) Differential effects of anxiolytic and non-anxiolytic benzodiazepine receptor ligands on performance of a differential reinforcement of low rate (DRL) schedule. *Behav Pharmacol* 5: 4–14

39 Griebel G, Sanger DJ, Perrault G (1996) Further evidence for differences between non-selective and BZ-1 (ω1) selective, benzodiazepine receptor ligands in murine models of "state" and "trait" anxiety. *Neuropharmacology* 35: 1081–1091

40 Griebel G, Sanger DJ, Perrault G (1996) The Mouse Defense Test Battery: Evaluation of the effects of non-selective and BZ-1 (ω1) selective, benzodiazepine receptor ligands. *Behav Pharmacol* 7: 560–572

41 Griebel G, Perrault G, Sanger DJ (1998) Limited anxiolytic-like effects of non-benzodiazepine hypnotics in rodents. *J Psychopharmacol* 12: 356–365

42 Rudolph U, Crestani F, Benke D, Martin JR, Benson JA, Keist R, Fritschy J-M, Löw K, Blüthmann H, Mohler H (1998) Function of GABA$_A$-receptor subtypes: mice with point-mutated

diazepam-insensitive GABA$_A$ α_1-receptors. *Soc Neurosci Abstr* 24: 1990

43 Griebel G, Perrault G, Letang V, Granger P, Avenet P, Schoemaker H, Sanger DJ (1999) New evidence that the pharmacological effects of benzodiazepine receptor ligands can be associated with activities at different BZ (ω) receptor subtypes. *Psychopharmacology* 146: 205–213

44 Pagot R, Cramer P, LHeritier C, Coquelin JP, Attali P (1993) Comparison of the efficacy and tolerability of zolpidem 20 mg and triazolam 0.5 mg in anxious or depressed insomniac patients. *Curr Ther Res Clin Exp* 53: 88–97

45 Ballenger JC, McDonald S, Noyes R, Rickels K, Sussman N, Woods S, Patin J, Singer J (1991) The first double-blind, placebo-controlled trial of a partial benzodiazepine agonist abecarnil (ZK 112-119) in generalized anxiety disorder. *Psychopharmacol Bull* 27: 171–179

46 Small GW, Bystritsky A (1997) Double-blind, placebo-controlled trial of two doses of abecarnil for geriatric anxiety. *J Clin Psychiat* 58 (Suppl. 11): 24–29

47 Lydiard RB, Ballenger JC, Rickels K (1997) A double-blind evaluation of the safety and efficacy of abecarnil, alprazolam, and placebo in outpatients with generalized anxiety disorder. Abecarnil Work Group. *J Clin Psychiat* 58 Suppl 11: 11–18

48 Lippa AS, Critchett D, Sano MC, Klepner CA, Greenblatt EN, Coupet J, Beer B (1979) Benzodiazepine receptors: cellular and behavioral characteristics. *Pharmacol Biochem Behav* 10: 831–843

49 Perrault G, Morel E, Sanger DJ, Zivkovic B (1990) Differences in pharmacological profiles of a new generation of benzodiazepine and non-benzodiazepine hypnotics. *Eur J Pharmacol* 187: 487–494

50 Stephens DN, Schneider HH, Kehr W, Jensen LH, Petersen E, Honore T (1987) Modulation of anxiety by β-carbolines and other benzodiazepine receptor ligands: relationship of pharmacological to biochemical measures of efficacy. *Brain Res* 19: 309–318

51 Turski L, Stephens DN, Jensen LH, Petersen EN, Meldrum BS, Patel S, Hansen JB, Loscher W, Schneider HH, Schmiechen R (1990) Anticonvulsant action of the β-carboline abecarnil: studies in rodents and baboon, Papio papio. *J Pharmacol Exp Ther* 253: 344–352

52 Zivkovic B, Morel E, Joly D, Perrault G, Sanger DJ, Lloyd KG (1990) Pharmacological and behavioral profile of alpidem as an anxiolytic. *Pharmacopsychiatry* 23 Suppl 3: 108–113

53 Thiebot MH (1985) Some evidence for amnesic-like effects of benzodiazepines in animals. *Neurosci Biobehav Rev* 9: 95–100

54 Sanger DJ, Joly D, Zivkovic B (1986) Effects of zolpidem, a new imidazopyridine hypnotic, on the acquisition of conditioned fear in mice: Comparison with triazolam and CL 218,872. *Psychopharmacology* 90: 207–210

55 Ozawa M, Sugimachi K, Nakada Kometani Y, Akai T, Yamaguchi M (1994) Chronic pharmacological activities of the novel anxiolytic β-carboline abecarnil in rats. *J Pharmacol Exp Ther* 269: 457–462

56 Sanger DJ, Benavides J, Perrault G, Morel E, Cohen C, Joly D, Zivkovic B (1994) Recent developments in the behavioral pharmacology of benzodiazepine (ω) receptors: Evidence for the functional significance of receptor subtypes. *Neurosci Biobehav Rev* 18: 355–372

57 Hege SG, Ellinwood EH, Wilson WH, Helligers CAM, Graham SM (1997) Psychomotor effects of the anxiolytic abecarnil: A comparison with lorazepam. *Psychopharmacology* 131: 101–107

58 Allen D, Curran H, V, Lader M (1993) The effects of single doses of CL284,846, lorazepam, and placebo on psychomotor and memory function in normal male volunteers. *Eur J Clin Pharmacol* 45: 313–320

59 Beer B, Ieni JR, Wu WM, Clody D, Amorusi P, Rose J, Mart T, Gaudreault J, Cato A, Stern W (1994) A placebo-controlled evaluation of single, escalating doses of CL 284,846, a non-benzodiazepine hypnotic. *J Clin Pharmacol* 34: 335–344

60 Colpaert FC, Niemegeers CJ, Janssen PA (1976) Theoretical and methodological considerations on drug discrimination learning. *Psychopharmacologia* 46: 169–177

61 Haug T, Gotestam KG (1982) Onset and offset of the diazepam stimulus complex. *Pharmacol Biochem Behav* 17: 1171–1174

62 Sanger DJ, Griebel G, Perrault G, Claustre Y, Schoemaker H (1999) Discriminative stimulus effects of drugs acting at GABA$_A$ receptors: differential profiles and receptor selectivity. *Pharmacol Biochem Behav* 64: 269–273

63 Sanger DJ, Benavides J (1993) Discriminative stimulus effects of ω (BZ) receptor ligands: Correlation with *in vivo* inhibition of [^{3}H]-flumazenil binding in different regions of the rat central nervous system. *Psychopharmacology* 111: 315–322

64 Hutchinson MA, Smith PF, Darlington CL (1996) The behavioural and neuronal effects of the chronic administration of benzodiazepine anxiolytic and hypnotic drugs. *Prog Neurobiol* 49: 73–97

65 Perrault G, Morel E, Sanger DJ, Zivkovic B (1993) Repeated treatment with alpidem, a new anxiolytic, does not induce tolerance or physical dependence. *Neuropharmacology* 32: 855–863

66 Sanger DJ, Zivkovic B (1987) Investigation of the development of tolerance to the actions of zolpidem and midazolam. *Neuropharmacology* 26: 1513–1518

67 Sanger DJ, Zivkovic B (1992) Differential development of tolerance to the depressant effects of benzodiazepine and non-benzodiazepine agonists at the ω (BZ) modulatory sites of $GABA_A$ receptors. *Neuropharmacology* 31: 693–700

68 Cohen C, Sanger DJ (1994) Effects of chronic treatment with triazolam on operant responding in rats. *Pharmacol Biochem Behav* 49: 455–461

69 Löscher W, Rundfeldt C, Honack D, Ebert U (1996) Long-term studies on anticonvulsant tolerance and withdrawal characteristics of benzodiazepine receptor ligands in different seizure models in mice. 2. The novel imidazoquinazolines NNC 14-0185 and NNC 14-0189. *J Pharmacol Exp Ther* 279: 573–581

70 VonVoigtlander PF, Lewis RA (1991) A rapid screening method for the assessment of benzodiazepine receptor-related physical dependence in mice. Evaluation of benzodiazepine-related agonists and partial agonists. *J Pharmacol Meth* 26: 1–5

71 Loscher W, Rundfeldt C, Honack D (1991) Tolerance to anticonvulsant effects of the partial benzodiazepine receptor agonist abecarnil in kindled rats involves learning. *Eur J Pharmacol* 202: 303–310

72 Sannerud CA, Ator NA, Griffiths RR (1992) Behavioral pharmacology of abecarnil in baboons: Self-injection, drug discrimination and physical dependence. *Behav Pharmacol* 3: 507–516

73 Serra M, Ghiani CA, Foddi MC, Galici R, Motzo C, Biggio G (1993) Failure of flumazenil to precipitate a withdrawal syndrome in cats chronically treated with the new anxioselective β-carboline derivative abecarnil. *Behav Pharmacol* 4: 529–533

74 Steppuhn KG, Schneider HH, Turski L, Stephens DN (1993) Long-term treatment with abecarnil does not induce diazepam-like dependence in mice. *J Pharmacol Exp Ther* 264: 1395–1400

75 Schlich D, Heritier C, Coquelin JP, Attali P, Kryrein HJ (1991) Long-term treatment of insomnia with zolpidem: a multicentre general practitioner study of 107 patients. *J Int Med Res* 19: 271–279

76 Herrmann WM, Kubicki ST, Boden S, Eich F, X, Attali P, Coquelin JP (1993) Pilot controlled double-blind study of the hypnotic effects of zolpidem in patients with chronic 'learned' insomnia: psychometric and polysomnographic evaluation. *J Int Med Res* 21: 306–322

77 Monti JM, Attali P, Monti D, Zipfel A, De La Giclais B, Morselli PL (1994) Zolpidem and rebound insomnia – A double-blind, controlled polysomnographic study in chronic insomniac patients. *Pharmacopsychiatry* 27: 166–175

78 Monti JM, Monti D, Estevez F, Giusti M (1996) Sleep in patients with chronic primary insomnia during long-term zolpidem administration and after its withdrawal. *Int Clin Psychopharmacol* 11: 255–263

79 Ware JC, Walsh JK, Scharf MB, Roehrs T, Roth T, Vogel GW (1997) Minimal rebound insomnia after treatment with 10-mg zolpidem. *Clin Neuropharmacol* 20: 116–125

80 Morton S, Lader M (1992) Alpidem and lorazepam in the treatment of patients with anxiety disorders: comparison of physiological and psychological effects. *Pharmacopsychiatry* 25: 177–181

81 Sakamoto T, Uchimura N, Mukai M, Mizuma H, Shirakawa S, I, Nakazawa Y (1998) Efficacy of L-846 in patients with insomnia: evaluation by polysomnography. *Psychiat Clin Neurosci* 52: 156–157

82 Aufdembrinke B (1998) Abecarnil, a new beta-carboline, in the treatment of anxiety disorders. *Brit J Psychiat* 173: 55–63

83 Pollack MH, Worthington JJ, Manfro GG, Otto MW, Zucker BG (1997) Abecarnil for the treatment of generalized anxiety disorder: a placebo-controlled comparison of two dosage ranges of abecarnil and buspirone. *J Clin Psychiat* 58 (Suppl. 11): 19–23

The 5-HT$_{1A}$ receptor: an unkept promise?

Louise R. Levine and William Z. Potter

Lilly Research Laboratories, Eli Lilly and Company, Lilly Corporate Center DC 1730, Indianapolis, IN 46285, USA

Introduction

Stimulation of 5-HT$_{1A}$ receptors appears to be the most plausible basis for the anxiolytic effects of buspirone and has been hypothesized to explain effects of SSRIs in depression and panic disorder [1]. A surprising number of relatively selective agonists have been developed since the introduction of buspirone (Mead Johnson) in 1986 for anxiety. Despite the plethora of preclinical models in which 5-HT$_{1A}$ agonists have produced evidence suggestive of anxiolytic *and* antidepressant activity, no new compound other than tandospirone (Sumitomo, Pfizer) has been registered. The large number of presentations at meetings, notations in industry media or corporate press releases, and much smaller number of peer reviewed publications on phase II/III studies underway in patients with generalized anxiety disorder or depression give a very mixed picture on these newer agents. Until the recent FDA approval of the antidepressant venlafaxine (Wyeth-Ayrst) (a mixed 5HT and noradrenergic uptake inhibitor at higher doses) for generalized anxiety disorder (GAD), there were no successors to buspirone or the benzodiazepines in the United States or Europe.

Early positive findings in anxiety with newer 5-HT$_{1A}$ agonists have not been followed by subsequent definitive data on efficacy. There are at least five explanations for the inconsistent data that arose from our evolving knowledge of the molecular pharmacology of 5-HT$_{1A}$ receptors in different species and clinical trial experience:

1) Efficacy is dependent on stimulating specific populations of 5-HT$_{1A}$ receptors (involving regional and pre- or postsynaptic localization) requiring a narrow concentration range, which varies within and across individuals according to the "state" of their serotonin system. If so, traditional clinical trials, which do not control for this possibility, would yield highly inconsistent results.
2) The pharmacodynamics of 5-HT$_{1A}$ agonism are such that individuals are either directly or subliminally aware of the presence of "active drug" and hence show effects over placebo [2].

3) Direct agonism on targets that show extensive down regulation may be intrinsically limited in maintaining sustained effects; interestingly, preclinical and clinical studies differ in their estimates of 5-HT$_{1A}$ down regulation [3, 4].

4) Where efficacy is seen, it is not due to 5-HT$_{1A}$ agonism itself but due to other actions such as α_2 adrenoreceptor antagonism by a metabolite (e.g. 1-(2-pyrimidinyl)-piperazine (1-PP) [5–7].

5) None of the tested compounds subsequent to buspirone achieves the "right" degree of agonism. According to this argument, if a compound had the critical degree of intrinsic efficacy it would show consistent results.

The last possibility is included for the sake of completeness to acknowledge an implicit or explicit point made in a number of reviews on the pharmacology of 5-HT$_{1A}$ receptors [3, 4]. This question of the right amount of agonism is also germane to understanding the first possibility 1 around which this critique is organized. Possibilities 2–4 are noted but do not emerge as likely reasons given what we present below. Knowledge of an extraordinarily complex distribution and regulation of 5-HT$_{1A}$ receptors in rodent and, to the extent evaluable in human brain continues to evolve [4, 5, 8, 9]. We will briefly highlight those complexities that make it so difficult to predict the effects of 5-HT$_{1A}$ agonists in living systems.

The 5-HT$_{1A}$ receptor is a member of the 5HT$_1$ receptor family with a high affinity for serotonin and coupled through G proteins to potassium channels or negatively to adenylate cyclase [3, 5, 10]. The highest density of receptor subtype is in the limbic system (e.g. hippocampus, septum, entorhinal cortex, and amygdala) where it is thought to play a role in emotional processes. 8-OH-DPAT is the classic selective agonist for the 5-HT$_{1A}$ receptor although recent studies reveal that even this ligand can behave as an antagonist under certain experimental conditions [5, 8]. Activation of this receptor in animals leads to such well-characterized physiological changes as hypothermia, which are easily quantified and provide multiple measures which to measure the activity of compounds [1, 4]. Studies of the preclinical neuropharmacology of buspirone (most generally regarded as a partial agonist) and related azaspirones went through several phases, the initial focus on effects in anti-anxiety models which it now appears are best explained by 5-HT$_{1A}$ partial agonism at presynaptic sites in contrast to a possible role of post-synaptic receptors in models of depression [4, 11]. Recent reviews on the biochemical and behavioral effects of 5-HT$_{1A}$ agonists with varying degrees of efficacy suggest that for depression compounds closer to full agonists may be better [4, 5, 8].

Given their complex pharmacology it is not surprising that finding appropriate clinical doses and concentrations of compounds with varying degrees of agonism has been difficult. Clinical pharmacological studies with more or less partial and full 5-HT$_{1A}$ agonists have yielded highly variable results across and within compounds [5] depending on whether one is looking at temperature, neuroendocrine, or behavioral responses. For instance, studies in healthy volunteers with ipsapirone (Bristol-Myers Squibb) agree on a hypothermic (presynaptic?) response [10] but vary with regard to ACTH, prolactin, and growth hormone changes (postsynaptic responses)[12]. These studies in healthy volunteer subjects, which are relatively easy to control, capture some of the variability in response to even a single compound and our lack of ability to pinpoint the mechanistic basis for the variability. Similarly, chronic administration to healthy subjects and/or patients of compounds known to affect serotonin function in humans (tricyclic antidepressants [TCAs] and SSRIs) produces some down-regulation of responses to 5-HT$_{1A}$ agonists (not predicted by preclinical models) but consistency with animal models only in terms of the hypothermic response [10]. As an example, Rausch et al. [3] showed increased cortisol levels after gepirone (Fabre-Kramer) administration to acutely depressed subjects but with attenuation of this effect following 3–6 weeks treatment suggesting desensitization after chronic administration. More recently it has been shown that chronic paroxetine (Smith Kline Beecham) (an SSRI) but not nefazedone (Bristol-Myers Squibb) (a 5HT$_2$ antagonist) attenuates endocrine and hypothermic responses to gepirone [13]. Thus although there appears to be at least one "well-defined" physiologic consequence of 5-HT$_{1A}$ stimulation (i.e. hypothermia) all other (objective) measures are highly variable although doses can be found that produce one or more endocrine responses [12].

For our review of the clinical literature of trials what has emerged as relatively consistent is the subjective side-effect profile of 5-HT$_{1A}$ agonists (dizziness, nausea, and headache), unfortunately at doses associated with apparent therapeutic efficacy. Interestingly, there is no obvious link between these side-effects and any objective pharmacological mechanism or physiologic effects (i.e. cardiovascular parameters do *not* change), or a presynaptic *vs.* postsynaptic site of action. It has been difficult if not impossible, to date, to find doses that separate "therapeutic" and "adverse" effects. With this background, we turn to a brief review of the current clinical status of compounds claimed to act primarily at the 5-HT$_{1A}$ receptor.

Methods

A search of the world's clinical literature on drugs acting primarily at the 5-HT$_{1A}$ receptor was carried using a number of databases: IMS R and D Focus, Pharma projects, ADIS R and D Insight, Investigational Drug Database (IDdb) which are compound-specific. In addition, we searched MEDLINE, Requestor, Profound, Dialog Pharma files and IMS Company Profiles.

Recent reviews have addressed the data on buspirone in both anxiety and depression [14–17]. In this review we focus on newer compounds with predominant activity at the 5-HT$_{1A}$ receptor while recognizing that numerous agents are also under development that combine agonism (or antagonism) at the 1A receptor with other actions.

5-HT$_{1A}$ compounds thought to still be under clinical development

Even restricting one's focus to agents selective for the 5-HT$_{1A}$ receptor, an incomplete list in 1997 included 15 agents at various stages of development [18]. There is insufficient non-proprietary data available to allow us to clearly determine the current status of most of these, especially with regard as to whether they are likely to ever reach the US or European markets. We have purposely omitted any discussion of ipsapirone since it was discontinued from further clinical development [19]. In Table 1 we have selected 12 compounds with the most published clinical data or those reported to be in Phase II/III clinical trials.

Table 1. Compounds active primarily at the 5-HT$_{1A}$ receptor believed to be targeted for anxiety

Compound (Company)	Published clinical data (Phase II/III)	Partial (P) or "full" (F) agonism; antagonist (A)	Clinical evidence for effectiveness in anxiety	Comments
Ipsapirone (Bayer)	Y	P	Y	Discontinued [19]
Gepirone (Fabre Kramer)	Y	P	Y	Thought to be submitted for registration [31]
Tandospirone (Sumitomo; Pfizer)	Y	P	Y	Registered in Japan only for treatment of anxiety disorders [32, 33]
Zalospirone (American Home Products)	Y	P	N	Current status unknown; reported only in depression
Flesinoxan (Solvay Duphar)	Y	F	Y	Current status unknown
Lesopitron (Esteve)	Y	P	N	Current status unknown
Bay-X-3702 (Bayer)	N	F?	unknown	Primarily targeted for neuroprotection [46-48] Current status unknown
MKC-242 (Mitsubishi Chemical)	N	F?	unknown	Current status unknown
S-15535 (Servier)	N	A	unknown	Current status unknown
Alnespirone (Servier)	N	F	unknown	Current status unknown
Sunepitron (CP-93393) (Pfizer)	N	F	unknown	Current status unknown
DU-125530 (Solvay Duphar BV)	N	F	unknown	Current status unknown

Gepirone, a pyridinyl piperazine azaspirone acts as a full agonist *in vivo* at presynaptic 5-HT$_{1A}$ autoreceptors, but as a partial agonist at postsynaptic 5-HT$_{1A}$ autoreceptors in brain limbic structures [20] and has been so classified in the table. Its actions appear similar to those of buspirone except for greater selectivity for 5-HT$_{1A}$ receptors over dopamine D$_2$ receptors [20]. Based on preclinical data there is a possibility of α_2-adrenoreceptor activity of gepirone (similar to that of ipsapirone) mediated by the common metabolite 1-PP although there is no evidence that sufficient concentrations are achieved in humans to produce these effects [21].

Interestingly, despite its classification as a partial agonist at post-synaptic receptors, a number of small studies [21] as well as larger Phase II/III studies [22–24] have shown efficacy for this compound in major depressive disorder including atypical depression [25]. Additionally, and in keeping with its preclinical profile, there have been trials in anxiety disorders including panic and generalized anxiety. In an open 6-week panic disorder study, 11/17 evaluable patients showed improvement by 6 weeks as measured by several scales [26]. More impressively, a study of 198 patients with GAD who received diazepam, gepirone, or placebo in escalating dosages revealed a delayed anxiolytic effect for gepirone [27], similar to results seen in prior studies with buspirone.

Bristol-Myers Squibb terminated its activity with this compound for undisclosed reasons and licensed it to Fabre-Kramer, which apparently continues Phase III testing with gepirone [28–30]. The "Pink Sheet" reported the filing of a New Drug Application (NDA) in 1996, but this compound has yet to be registered [31].

Tandospirone, launched in Japan in 1996 for anxiety [32, 33], shares common pharmacological features with other compounds from the azaspirone class. It demonstrates similar affinity to the 5-HT$_{1A}$ receptors as does buspirone acting as a full agonist at presynaptic sites, a partial agonist at postsynaptic sites, and showing low affinity for the dopamine D$_2$ receptor [32, 33]. Although the results of some early clinical trials were published in the Japanese literature earlier this decade [32, 24], no placebo-controlled clinical trials have been published in the English literature. Summaries of these studies suggest a similar efficacy/safety profile to other 5-HT$_{1A}$ receptor ligands. The side-effect profile includes headache, dizziness, and nausea like that reported for other 5-HT$_{1A}$ agonists [32]. This compound apparently failed to show sufficient activity in the clinic for the treatment of depression but is reportedly in Phase III for GAD in the US [32].

Flesinoxan (Solvay Duphar BV) acts as a full agonist at the presynaptic somatodendritic 5-HT$_{1A}$ receptors and like 8-OH-DPAT, may also act as a partial agonist at postsynaptic receptors [35] despite earlier characterization as a full agonist. We have maintained this earlier characterization as a full agonist in Table 1 since it is the closest to meeting this criterion. Unlike the azaspirones, flesinoxan is not metabolized into 1-PP. Whether this lack of metabolism is relevant to distinguishing it from the other compounds in terms of clinical effects remains to be seen. Overall, flesinoxan represents one of the "cleanest" compounds to date for assessing the potential of full or close to full 5-HT$_{1A}$ agonism.

An early study exploring flesinoxan as a probe of 5-HT$_{1A}$ function in healthy male subjects, demonstrated dose-dependent complaints of light-headedness and nausea [36]. Although as noted in the Introduction, one might have targeted a full agonist to depression, available published information on flesinoxan is in anxiety. In a five-arm GAD study comparing three dose levels of flesinoxan to placebo and alprazolam, both the highest dose and alprazolam showed significant separation from placebo in terms of HAM-A change from baseline [37]. Unfortunately, two pilot studies in panic disorder [38] showed a worsening of the disorder or no effect but with increased anxiety reported, perhaps reflecting its potency as a likely full agonist. The lack of further published clinical information on this molecule may indicate that flesinoxan failed to meet its preclinical and early clinical expectations as either an antidepressant or an anxiolytic.

Another azaspirone partial agonist, zalospirone (American Home Products), is thought to have greater affinity for presynaptic, autodendritic receptors [39] which might suggest greater activity in anxiety disorders. Interestingly, this compound has only been studied in patients with major depression and is notable for the finding that about half of the patients had withdrawn as a result of adverse events by the end of the study [39, 40]. The current fate of this compound is unknown.

Yet another azaspirone partial agonist, lesopitron (Esteve), *is* reported to be in Phase II trials for anxiety disorders [41, 42]. Sramek et al. [43] carried out a bridging study in patients with anxiety to determine the maximum tolerated dose instead of selecting doses on the basis of findings in healthy volunteers. Nonetheless, similar to other 5-HT$_{1A}$ agonists, lesopitron-associated adverse effects included headache, dizziness, and nausea [42]. We were unable to identify any further published clinical studies.

Several additional compounds for which we could find no published clinical data but which the "pipeline" sources list as currently under active Phase II or III investigation in anxiety disorders include the following:

- MKC242 (Mitsubishi Chemical), thought to exhibit full and partial agonism at pre- and postsynaptic 5-HT$_{1A}$ receptors respectively, reported to be in Phase II [44, 45];
- Repinotan (BAY-X-3702) (Bayer AG), a novel aminomethylchroman derivative, thought to be in phase II/III for acute ischemic stroke and traumatic brain injury but unknown if being pursued for anxiety [46–48]. Like other 5-HT$_{1A}$ agonists this compound also produced headache, dizziness, and nausea during Phase I studies [49];
- Sunepitron (CP-93393) (Pfizer), thought to be in Phase II or III as an anxiolytic and/or antidepressant [50, 51];
- DU-125530 (Solvay Duphar BV), a 5-HT$_{1A}$ *antagonist* thought to be in Phase II trials for anxiety [52, 53];

- S-15535 and alnespirone (S20499) (Servier), reportedly in Phase II clinical trials in France as anxiolytics [54–57].

It is worth noting that DU-125530 is reported to be an *antagonist*, reflecting the fact that in some animal models 5-HT$_{1A}$ antagonism shows anxiolytic activity [1, 9]. This raises an additional range of questions regarding our limited understanding of 5-HT$_{1A}$ function, which are beyond the scope of this chapter.

Conclusion

Many reports on the activity of 5-HT$_{1A}$ agonists suggested great promise in terms of treating anxiety and affective disorders [8, 15, 58, 59]. The partial list of more recent compounds acting primarily at this receptor previously or currently in development reflects the intense research effort over the past two decades. Do the newer drugs of this class of compounds actually possess a significant degree of novelty that separates them in either efficacy (including an extension of indications) or safety from buspirone? The available data would argue no.

There do appear to be preclinical "advantages" in terms of selectivity and potency that, in some quarters, may be interpreted as limiting partial agonists to anxiety and full agonists to depression. Animal studies, however, show a range of receptor occupancy as well as "efficacy" depending on multiple pre-existing factors that cannot be controlled in clinical studies [4, 5, 8]. Postsynaptic 5-HT$_{1A}$ mediated-effects in the hippocampus or other areas (e.g. vestibular area) might be the site for a major pharmacological effect. Could this be the basis for the subjectively and commonly reported "dizziness" or "lightheadedness" in the absence of objective findings? Furthermore, clinical evidence from published literature, and what can be deduced by the high failure rate at all phases of development, suggests that this characteristic may limit the commercial success of 5-HT$_{1A}$ agonists. Moreover, the available data do not suggest that partial *vs.* full agonism confers any relative advantage or disadvantage in terms of anxiety or depression. The only hint that these distinctions are clinically relevant derives from the apparent worsening of panic symptoms after administration of flesinoxan, identified as a full agonist.

Thus, this myriad of compounds shows seemingly few differentiating attributes from buspirone except perhaps greater specificity at the receptor site. Despite a few encouraging published reports of Phase III studies with gepirone, this pharmacological class fails to live up to its preclinical promise of safer and more effective anxiolytics (and antidepressants). The cost of the preclinical research alone has been enormous and that of all cumulative clinical studies must be in excess of a billion dollars! Given the additional issues of 1) highly variable placebo response rates in both anxiety and depression trials; 2) a move towards larger and larger studies pursuing smaller and smaller effect sizes; and 3) an apparent narrow therapeutic index; further pursuit of selective 5-HT$_{1A}$ agonists as monotherapy for anxiety (and depression) may be unwarranted.

Acknowledgements
The authors wish to thank the following: Pam Kiser, Kathryn Lavengood, and Beverly Pierce, for all of their assistance in gathering information regarding the status of 5-HT$_{1A}$ receptors which are currently or no longer under clinical investigation; and Dr. Peter Bieck for his technical assistance in compiling relevant pharmacological references about the 5-HT$_{1A}$ receptor.

References

1 Rasmussen K, Rocco VP (1995) Recent progress in serotonin. *In*: JA Briston (ed.): *Ann Reports in Medicinal Chemistry, Vol 30*, Academic Press, New York, 1–9

2 Enserink M (1999) Can placebo be the cure? *Science* 284: 238–240

3 Rausch JL, Stahl SM, Hauger RL (1990) Cortisol and growth hormone responses to the 5-HT$_{1A}$ agonists gepirone in depressed patients. *Biol Psychiat* 28: 73–78

4 Fletcher A, Cliffe IA, Dourish CT (1993) Silent 5-HT$_{1A}$ receptor antagonists: utility as research tools and therapeutic agents. *Trends Pharmacol Sci* 14: 441–448

5 DeVry J (1995) 5-HT$_{1A}$ receptor agonists: recent developments and controversial issues. *Psychopharmacology* 121: 1–26

6 Blier P, Curet O, Chaput Y, de Montigny C (1991) Tandospirone and its metabolite, 1-(2-pyrimidil)-piperazine, II: effects of acute administration of 1-PP and long-term administration of tandospirone on noradrenergic neurotransmission. *Neuropharmacology* 30: 691–701

7 Gobbi M, Frittoli E, Mennini T (1990) Antagonist properties of 1-(2-pyrimidil)-piperazine at presynaptic adrenoceptors in the rat brain. *Eur J Pharmacol* 180: 183–186

8 Borsini F (1998) Pharmacology of 5-HT$_{1A}$ receptors: critical aspects. *CNS Spectrums* 3: 17–38

9 Kenakin T (1987) Agonists, partial agonists, antagonists, inverse agonists and agonist/antagonists? *Trends Pharmacol Sci* 8: 423–426

10 Gartside SE, Cowen PJ (1994) 5-HT$_{1A}$ receptors and antidepressant drug action. *In*: SA Montgomery and TH Corn (eds): *Psycopharmacology of depression*. Oxford University Press, Oxford, 66–86

11 Yocca FD (1990) Neurochemistry and neurophysiology of buspirone and gepirone: interactions at presynaptic and postsynaptic 5-HT$_{1A}$ receptors. *J Clin Psychopharmacol* 10: 6S–12S

12 Cleare AJ, Forsling M, Bond AJ (1998) Neuroendocrine and hypothermic effects of 5-HT$_{1A}$ receptor stimulation with ipsapirone in healthy men: a placebo-controlled study. *Int Clin Psychopharmacol* 13: 23–32

13 Sargent P, Williamson DJ, Pearson G, Odontiadis J, Cowen PJ (1997) Effect of paroxetine and nefazodone on 5-HT$_{1A}$ receptor sensitivity. *Psychopharmacology* 132: 296–302

14 Gammans RE, Stringfellow JC, Hvizdos AJ, Seidehamel RJ, Cohn JB, Wilcox CS, Fabre LF, Pecknold JC, Smith WT, Rickels K (1992) Use of buspirone in patients with generalized anxiety disorder and co-existing depressive symptoms: a meta-analysis of eight randomized, controlled studies. *Neuropsychobiology* 25: 193–201

15 Pecknold JC (1994) Serotonin 5-HT$_{1A}$ agonists: a comparative review. *CNS Drugs* 2: 234–251

16 Fulton B, Brogden RN (1997) Buspirone: an updated review of its clinical pharmacology and therapeutic applications. *CNS Drugs* 7: 68–88

17 Apter JT, Allen LA (1999) Buspirone: future directions. *J Clin Psychopharmacol* 19: 86–93

18 Griebel G (1997) Serotonergic drugs in animal models of anxiety: an update, Serotonin, vol. 2, no. 6. *In*: *The investigational drugs database* [Corporate Intranet]. © 1997–1998 Current Drugs Ltd. [1999, March 2]

19 IMSWorld Publications Editorial Staff Ipsapirone (pINN) Drug Abstract. *In*: *IMSWorld RandD Focus*, [Lotus Notes]. © 1999 IMSWorld Publications Limited. [30 March 1999]

20 IMSWorld Publications Editorial Staff Gepirone (INN) Drug Abstract. *In*: *IMSWorld RandD Focus*, [Lotus Notes]. © 1999 IMSWorld Publications Limited. [30 March 1999]

21 Drugs Editorial Staff. Gepirone Drug Report *In*: *The Investigational Drugs database*, [Lotus Notes]. © 1997–1998 Current Drugs Ltd. [30 March 1999]

22 Jenkins SW, Robinson DS, Fabre Jr LF, Andary JJ, Messina ME, Reich LA (1990) Gepirone in the treatment of major depression. *J Psychopharmacol* 10(s): 77–87

23 Wilcox CS, Ferguson JM, Dale JL, Heiser JF (1996) A double-blind trial of low- and high-dose ranges of gepirone-ER compared with placebo in the treatment of depressed outpatients. *Psychopharmacol Bull* 32: 335–342

24 Feiger AD (1996) A double-blind comparison of gepirone extended release, imipramine, and placebo in the treatment of outpatient major depression. *Psychopharmacol Bull* 32: 659–665

25 McGrath PJ, Stewart JW, Quitkin FM, Wager S, Jenkins SW, Archibald DG, Stringfellow JC, Robinson DS (1994) Gepirone treatment of atypical depression: preliminary evidence of serotonergic involvement. *J Clin Psychopharmacol* 14: 347–352

26 Pecknold JC, Luthe L, Scott Fluery M-H, Jenkins S (1993) Gepirone and the treatment of panic disorder: an open study. *J Clin Psychopharmacol* 13: 145–149

27 Rickels K, Schweizer E, DeMartinis N, Mandos L, Mercer C (1997) Gepirone and diazepam in generalized anxiety disorder: a placebo-controlled trial. *J Clin Psychopharmacol* 17: 272–277

28 Bristol-Myers Squibb (1993) Licensing Information. *Company Communication* September 10

29 International Editorial Staff Gepirone (BMY 13805, MJ 13805) Profile *In: Adis R and D Insight*, [Lotus Notes]. © 1998 Adis International Ltd. [30 March 1999]

30 PBJ Publications Editorial Staff Pharmaprojects Record No.: 006405. *In: PJB Pharmaprojects*, [Corporate Intranet]. © 1998 PJB Publications Ltd. [30 March 1999]

31 Fabre-Kramer gepirone NDA for depression under preparation (1996) *FDC Reports Pink Sheet* 58: 40 Tand G-10

32 Drugs Editorial Staff Tandospirone Drug Report. *In: The Investigational Drugs database*, [Lotus Notes]. © 1997–1998 Current Drugs Ltd. [30 March 1999]

33 Adis International Editorial Staff Tandospirone (Metanopirone, SM 3997, Sediel) *Profile In: Adis R and D Insight*, [Lotus Notes]. © 1998 Adis International Ltd. [30 March 1999]

34 Murasaki M, Mori A, Kudo Y (1993) Efficacy of a new anxiolytic, tandospirone (SM-3997) on neurosis. *Neuropsychopharmacology* 9 (Suppl): 125

35 Hadrav V, Blier P, Dennis T, Ortemann C, de Montigny C (1995) Characterization of 5-hydroxytryptamine 1A properties of flesinoxan: *in vivo* electrophysiology and hypothermia study. *Neuropharmacology* 34: 1311–1326

36 Seletti B, Bemkelfat C, Blier P, Annable L, Gilbert F, de Montigny C (1995) Serotonin 1A receptor activation by flesinoxan in humans: body temperature and neuroendocrine responses. *Neuropsychopharmacology* 13: 93–104

37 Bradford LD, Stevens G (1994) Double-blind, placebo controlled fixed dose study of flesinoxan in generalized anxiety disorder. *Amer Coll Neuropsychopharmacol* 167

38 van Vliet IM, Westenberg HGM, den Boer JA (1996) Effects of the 5-HT$_{1A}$ receptor agonist flesinoxan in panic disorder. *Psychopharmacology* 127: 174–180

39 Current Drugs Editorial Staff Zalospirone Drug Report. *In: The Investigational Drugs database*, [Lotus Notes]. © 1997–1998 Current Drugs Ltd. [14 April 1999]

40 Rickels K, Derivan A, Kunz N, Pally A, Schweizer E (1996) Zalospirone in major depression: a placebo-controlled multicenter study. *J Clin Psyhcopharmacol* 16: 212–217

41 Adis International Editorial Staff Lesopitron (E 4424) Profile. *In: Adis R and D Insight*, [Lotus Notes]. © 1998 Adis International Ltd. [30 March 1999]

42 Current Drugs Editorial Staff Lesopitron Drug Report. *In: The Investigational Drugs database*, [Lotus Notes]. © 1997–1998 Current Drugs Ltd. [30 March 1999]

43 Sramek JJ, Fresquet A, Marion-Lanais G, Hourani J, Jhee SS, Martinez L, Jensen CM, Bolles K, Carrington AT, Cutler NR (1996) Establishing the maximum tolerated dose of lesopitron in patients with generalized anxiety disorder: a bridging study. *J Clin Psychopharmacol* 16: 454–458

44 Adis International Editorial Staff MKC 242 Profile *In: Adis R and D Insight*, [Lotus Notes]. © 1998 Adis International Ltd. [30 March 1999]

45 Current Drugs Editorial Staff MKC-242 Drug Report. *In: The Investigational Drugs database*, [Lotus Notes]. © 1997–1998 Current Drugs Ltd. [30 March 1999]

46 Adis International Editorial Staff BAY X 3702 (BAY 3702) Profile *In: Adis R and D Insight*, [Lotus Notes]. © 1998 Adis International Ltd. [30 March 1999]

47 Current Drugs Editorial Staff Bay-x-3702 Drug Report *In: The Investigational Drugs database*, [Lotus Notes]. © 1997–1998 Current Drugs Ltd. [30 March 1999]

48 PBJ Publications Editorial Staff Pharmaprojects Record No.: 008383024493 *In: PJB Pharmaprojects*, [Corporate Intranet]. © 1998 PJB Publications Ltd. [30 March 1999]

49 De Vry J, Dietrich H, Glasser T (1997) BAY x 3702. *Drugs of the Future* 22: 341–349
50 Adis International Editorial Staff Sunepitron (CP 93393) Profile. *In: Adis R and D Insight*, [Lotus Notes]. © 1998 Adis International Ltd. [30 March 1999]
51 Current Drugs Editorial Staff Sunepitron Hydrochloride Drug Report *In: The Investigational Drugs database*, [Lotus Notes]. © 1997–1998 Current Drugs Ltd. [30 March 1999]
52 Current Drugs Editorial Staff DU-125530 Drug Report *In: The Investigational Drugs database*, [Lotus Notes]. © 1997–1998 Current Drugs Ltd. [30 March 1999]
53 PBJ Publications Editorial Staff Pharmaprojects Record No.: 027926 *In: PJB Pharmaprojects*, [Corporate Intranet]. © 1998 PJB Publications Ltd. [30 March 1999]
54 Adis International Editorial Staff S 15535 Profile *In: Adis R and D Insight*, [Lotus Notes]. © 1998 Adis International Ltd. [1 April 1999]
55 Current Drugs Editorial Staff S-15535 Drug Report *In: The Investigational Drugs database*, [Lotus Notes]. © 1997–1998 Current Drugs Ltd. [1 April 1999]
56 Adis International Editorial Staff Alnespirone (S 20499) Profile *In: Adis R and D Insight*, [Lotus Notes]. © 1998 Adis International Ltd. [30 March 1999]
57 Current Drugs Editorial Staff Alnespirone Drug Report *In: The Investigational Drugs database*, [Lotus Notes]. © 1997–1998 Current Drugs Ltd. [30 March 1999]
58 Ennis MD (1993) The therapeutic potential of 5-HT$_{1A}$ agonists *Curr Opin Invest Drugs* 2: 271–279
59 Heiser JF, Wilcox CS (1998) Serotonin 5-HT$_{1A}$ receptor agonists as antidepressants: pharmacological rationale and evidence for efficacy *CNS Drugs* 10: 343–353

5-HT$_{1B/D}$ receptors in anxiety

Chantal Moret

Les Grèzes, La Verdarié, 81100 Castres, France

Introduction

The last 30 years have seen the virtual monopoly of the anxiolytic market by benzodiazepines and more recently by the compounds which constitute the first part of this book. Among other neurotransmitters potentially involved in anxiety, serotonin (5-hydroxytryptamine, 5-HT) of course has a very prominent place. The neuropharmacology of 5-HT has been fundamentally revised in recent years with the discovery of multiple serotonin receptor subtypes [1].

According to the classification by Hartig et al. [2] based on molecular biology data, 5-HT$_{1B}$ receptors are found in high densities in substantia nigra, globus pallidus, striatum and basal ganglia [3], where they function as presynaptic inhibitory autoreceptors on serotonergic nerve terminals [4–14]. Other 5-HT$_{1B}$ receptors are located, as heteroreceptors, on other (non-serotonergic) nerve endings where they regulate the release of various neurotransmitters, while yet others may be situated postsynaptically on the target neurons of 5-HT projections [15, 16] (Fig. 1).

The 5-HT$_{1D}$ receptor codistributes with the 5-HT$_{1B}$ receptor in many brain regions and also seems to provide both autoreceptor and heteroreceptor functions [17]. The density of mRNA and receptor protein for the 5-HT$_{1D}$ receptor appears to be much lower than that of the closely related 5-HT$_{1B}$ receptor, which has made it difficult to separately evaluate the role of the 5-HT$_{1D}$ receptor [18]. Therefore much confusion has existed and still exists in the literature regarding the pharmacology and nomenclature of these 5-HT$_{1B}$ and 5-HT$_{1D}$ subtypes [19].

The lack of selective agonists and antagonists for 5-HT$_{1B}$ and 5-HT$_{1D}$ receptors has made it difficult to determine the neurochemical, behavioral or clinical effects controlled by these receptors. By combining data from various compounds with different receptor affinity profiles, however, it is possible to make a tentative assignment as to those effects which result from interactions at the 5-HT$_{1B}$ and 5-HT$_{1D}$ receptors.

In this chapter the neuropharmacology of the 5-HT$_{1B/D}$ receptor subtype is treated with the attempt to identify its possible functions and potential impli-

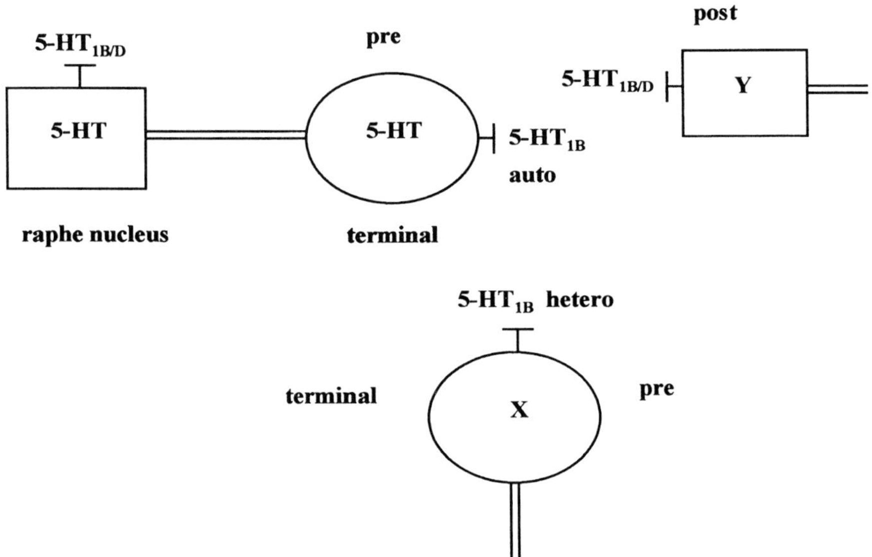

Figure 1. Schematic representation of the location of 5-HT$_{1B/D}$ receptors in brain. Rectangles represent cell bodies of neurons and ellipses represent terminals. X and Y are neurotransmitters (non serotonin). Pre is the presynaptic site and post is the postsynaptic site of the synapse. Auto: autoreceptor. Hetero: heteroreceptor.

cations in anxiety by the studies of associating the measurement of release and synthesis of serotonin and behavior.

Regulation of serotonin release

Receptors of the 5-HT$_{1B}$ subtype in animal and human brain have been shown to have an autoreceptor function regulating the release of serotonin [14, 12] (see above). These receptors are involved in a negative feedback mechanism through which the neurotransmitter, serotonin, can regulate its own release. They are located on neuronal terminals but their presence has also been shown at the level of the raphe nucleus [20–23] (Fig. 1) at least in some parts [13, 24] (see below).

Numerous studies have clearly shown that the neurotransmission of 5-HT is increased under acute stressful conditions [25, 26]. Bolaños-Jimenez et al. [27] have studied the possible effects of acute restraint (40 min) on the functional properties of 5-HT$_{1B}$ autoreceptors in the rat hippocampus by using the 5-HT$_{1B}$ receptor agonist 3-(1,2,5,6-tetrahydropyrid-4-yl)pyrolol[3,2,6]pyrid-5-one (CP-93,129). They have shown that the efficacy of this compound in inhibiting *in vitro* the K$^+$-evoked release of [^{3}H]5-HT is reduced in stressed rats as compared to naïve animals. Similarly, the responsiveness of 5-HT$_{1B}$ receptors inhibiting the release of [^{3}H]acetylcholine (presynaptic 5-HT$_{1B}$ heteroreceptors), is diminished by restraint. As stress is thought to be a causal factor for the etiology of anxiety, these interesting results support the potential involvement of 5-HT$_{1B}$ receptor dysfunction in the development of this psychiatric disorder.

The direct, *in vivo*, study of 5-HT autoreceptor function has become more accessible since the advent of intracerebral microdialysis, a technique which allows direct *in vivo* sampling and measurement of neurotransmitters and their metabolites in the extracellular fluid of different regions of the brain [28] of anaesthetized or freely moving animals.

CP-93,129, a 5-HT$_{1B}$ receptor agonist with about 100-fold higher affinity for 5-HT$_{1B}$ than for 5-HT$_{1A}$ binding sites [29], when administered *via* the dialysis perfusion medium, has been shown to cause a reduction of 5-HT output in the hippocampus of anaesthetized rats [30]. This effect was significantly antagonized by co-infusion of the non-selective 5-HT autoreceptor antagonist, methiothepin.

In the rat hypothalamus, methiothepin, when applied locally *via* the microdialysis probe, increased the extracellular levels of 5-HT both in the absence and in the presence of the 5-HT uptake inhibitor, citalopram, suggesting that in awake animals 5-HT autoreceptors in the terminal projection areas are tonically activated and exert a potent inhibitory tone on the release of 5-HT [31].

Guinea pigs are suitable animals to study terminal 5-HT$_{1B}$ autoreceptors since their receptors have a similar pharmacology to those in humans [32]. Local (*via* microdialysis probe) administration of the 5-HT$_{1A/B}$ agonist, 5-CT, into the frontal cortex of the freely moving guinea pig decreased extracellular 5-HT levels [33]. Sumatriptan, a 5-HT$_{1B/D}$ agonist, when added to the perfusion medium, similarly reduces extracellular levels of 5-HT in the frontal cortex of anaesthetized guinea pigs [34, 35] presumably *via* an activation of 5-HT$_{1B}$ autoreceptors. In guinea pig hypothalamus and dorsal raphe nucleus, local, through the probe administration of naratriptan, which is somewhat more selective for 5-HT$_{1B/D}$ receptors compared to 5-HT$_{1A}$ receptors than sumatriptan, also decreases the extracellular levels of 5-HT, an effect which is attenuated by the non-selective 5-HT$_1$ receptor antagonist, methiothepin at 1 μM, a concentration which does not modify by itself the outflow of 5-HT [36]. In guinea pig frontal cortex sumatriptan-induced inhibition of 5-HT release has been shown to be reversed by the 5-HT$_{1B}$ receptor antagonist, SB-224289 (2,3,6,7-tetrahydro-1'-methyl-5-{2'-methyl-4'-[(5-methyl-1, 2, 4-oxadiazole-3-yl)biphenyl-4-yl]carbonyl}Furo[2, 3-F]-indole-3-spiro-4'-piperidine oxalate [37]. The extracellular levels of 5-HT measured by microdialysis in hypothalamus of freely moving guinea pigs are increased by methiothepin when the concentrations of 10–100 μM are used [36]. Similarly, *in vivo* microdialysis measurements in guinea pig hypothalamus show a prolonged increase in extracellular levels of 5-HT following s.c. administration with the 5-HT$_{1D}$ receptor antagonist, CP-291,952 [38]. This suggests that, as in the rat, in the hypothalamus of freely moving guinea pig 5-HT autoreceptors are tonically activated and exert a potent inhibitory tone on the release of 5-HT. When this inhibition is removed by an antagonist, such as methiothepin, there is a major increase in 5-HT release. A similar effect has been found with methiothepin in guinea pig substantia nigra [39].

More recently, Roberts et al. [24] have proposed a new hypothesis concerning the distribution of $5\text{-HT}_{1B/D}$ autoreceptors. In the frontal cortex and striatum which are mainly dorsal raphe nucleus innervated areas, GR 127935 (N-[4-methoxy-3-(4-methyl-1-piperizinyl)phenyl]-2'-methyl-4'-(5-methyl-1,2,4-oxadiazole-3-yl)[1, 1'-biphenyl]-carboxamide), a $5\text{-HT}_{1B/D}$ receptor antagonist, acutely administered, decreases extracellular levels of 5-HT. The authors explain this decrease by antagonism of inhibitory $5\text{-HT}_{1B/D}$ receptors on raphe cell bodies, leading to a local increase in 5-HT, which, in turn, stimulates 5-HT_{1A} receptors to decrease cell firing, and hence 5-HT release from terminals. In contrast, the 5-HT_{1B} receptor antagonist, SB-224289, has no effect on 5-HT levels in either region. In the dentate gyrus, a region principally innervated by the median raphe nucleus, GR 127935 and SB-224289 increase extracellular levels of 5-HT, result suggesting a lack of $5\text{-HT}_{1B/D}$ receptors in the median raphe nucleus [24].

All these studies point out the complexity of the control of 5-HT neurotransmission and the role of 5-HT autoreceptors modulating the release of 5-HT is not as simple as expected a few years ago.

In spite of that complexity it has been successfully demonstrated by Rex et al. [40) that 5-HT_{1B} receptors are involved in cortical extracellular 5-HT release in guinea pigs on exposure to the elevated plus maze. Non-handled guinea pigs remain in a state of reflexive freezing for the entire 20 min observation period when subjected to the aversive conditions of the X-maze [41]. However, guinea pigs handled twice a day from birth do not exhibit reflexive freezing on exposure to the X-maze but show similar behaviour to that of rats [42, 43]. Under these aversive conditions of exposure to the elevated plus maze, the release of extracellular 5-HT is increased, an effect abolished by the non-selective 5-HT_1 receptor agonist, 5-carboxamidotryptamine (5-CT). Pretreatment with the selective 5-HT_{1B} receptor antagonist, GR 127935, antagonizes the effect of 5-CT on the aversion-induced increase in extracellular 5-HT on exposure to the elevated plus maze. These results indicate that the 5-HT_{1B} autoreceptor in the frontal cortex is functionally active under averse conditions. However some more work is needed to establish with certainty in which direction, pro- or anti-anxiety, it plays in this role.

5-HT-moduline is an endogenous peptide (tetrapeptide Leu-Ser-Ala-Leu, LSAL) characterized by its binding to 5-HT_{1B} receptors in the brain areas in which it is released. So, by inducing structural changes in these receptors, this peptide prevents 5-HT binding, thereby desensitizing the receptors and inhibiting serotonergic function [44]. As already mentioned above, several experimental studies showed that an acute stress, which is assumed to induce anxiety, increases 5-HT release in various brain areas, as measured by microdialysis [45–48]. Bolaños et al. [27] have shown that 5-HT_{1B} receptors are desensitized following an acute immobilization stress, and Seguin et al. [49] have shown that rats receiving 5-HT-moduline *via* intracerebroventricular injection exhibit a similar desensitization of their 5-HT$_{1B}$ receptors. In rats subjected to the acute immobilization stress, a major increase of 5-HT-moduline tissue content is observed in various brain areas. These researchers hypothesized that an excess of 5-HT-moduline induces a desensitization of 5-HT$_{1B}$ receptors, resulting in an excess of 5-HT activity which has been proposed to be closely related to anxiety. Therefore, even if one cannot yet understand the exact way of its action, 5-HT-moduline is likely to be involved in the pathophysiology of anxiety.

Even if there are not yet many studies associating the investigation of the function of the terminal autoreceptor and behaviour of stress or anxiety, it is highly probable that, by means of the microdialysis technique, future experiments will support and strenghthen the involvement of the terminal 5-HT$_{1B}$ autoreceptor dysfunction in the development of anxiety.

Regulation of serotonin synthesis

It is well established that activation of the somatodendritic 5-HT$_{1A}$ autoreceptors decrease 5-HT neuronal firing and, in turn, the synthesis, metabolism and release of the transmitter. Recently, however, studies in the rat [50] have shown that the 5-HT$_{1B/2C}$ receptor agonist, TFMPP (m-trifluoromethyl-phenylpiperazine), suppresses 5-HT synthesis *in vivo* as estimated by the accumulation of 5-hydroxytryptophan (5-HTP) after the inhibition of the amino acid decarboxylase, i.e. an index of tryptophan hydroxylation [51]. This suppression, which is evident in terminal projection areas such as the limbic forebrain and striatum, is also observed in axotomized animals, indicating that it is independent of neuronal firing [50]. Furthermore, a similar inhibitory effect of TFMPP on 5-HT synthesis is found *in vitro* in slice preparations in the presence of depolarizing concentrations of potassium. *In vitro* the effect of TFMPP is attenuated by the non-selective 5-HT receptor antagonist, methiothepin, as well as the 5-HT$_{1B}$ receptor antagonists, propranolol or cyanopindolol [50]. By comparison, the decrease of 5-HT synthesis in forebrain regions induced *in vivo* by 8-OH-DPAT is prevented by transection of the brain. In addition, 8-OH-DPAT does not decrease 5-HT synthesis *in vitro* [50]. These data thus suggest that the reduction of rat brain 5-HT synthesis by TFMPP is mediated by 5-HT autoreceptors located on the serotonergic axon terminals, and that this is a direct effect, independent of 5-HT neuronal firing [50].

This finding confirms earlier suggestions. For example, in one study using a similar *ex vivo* protocol [52, 53], systemically administered methiothepin was found to increase the synthesis of 5-HT in rat frontal cortex, while the 5-HT$_{1A/2}$ receptor antagonist, spiperone, has no effect thus suggesting the possible involvement of 5-HT$_{1B}$ autoreceptors in the modulation of 5-HT synthesis.

In guinea pig brain, systemic administration of GR 127935, a reportedly selective 5-HT$_{1B/D}$ receptor antagonist [54] increases 5-HT synthesis in the frontal cortex (maximum effect 233% of control). Smaller, but significant increases (55–60%) in 5-HT synthesis have also been found in other regions such as the hypothalamus, hippocampus and substantia nigra following systemic administration of similar doses of GR 127935 [36].

Recently it has been reported by Tingley et al. [38] that the high affinity 5-HT$_{1D}$ receptor antagonist CP-291,952 produces increases in 5-HT turnover (ratio of 5-HIAA/5-HT) in guinea pig cortex and other brain regions following oral administration and reverses the decrease in 5-HT turnover caused by the 5-HT$_{1D}$ receptor agonist CP-135,807 (3-(N-methylpyrrolidin-2R-yl-methyl)-5-(3-nitropyrid-2-ylamino)-1H-indole) in these regions.

Taken together, these findings observed in both rat and guinea pig strongly suggest that the terminal 5-HT$_{1B/D}$ autoreceptors can play a role in the regulation of 5-HT synthesis.

The studies associating stress or anxiety and measurement of 5-HT synthesis are not numerous. However, Chaouloff et al. [55] have used the Wistar-Kyoto (WKY) rat strain which displays high emotivity (e.g. anxiety) in stressful environments to assess the neurochemical bases of emotivity in comparison to Wistar rats. They observed that WKY rats, when compared with Wistar rats, display a lower hyperlocomotor response to the acute administration of the non-selective 5-HT receptor compound, RU 24969. Since RU 24969-induced hyperlocomotion has been proposed to be a postsynaptic 5-HT$_{1B}$ receptor-mediated response in rats [56, 57], they examined whether such a genetic difference in a 5-HT$_{1B}$ receptor-mediated response extends to 5-HT$_{1B}$ receptor-mediated function such as the inhibition of 5-HT synthesis at serotonergic nerve terminals [58, 50]. In the midbrain the accumulation of 5-HTP is higher in WKY rats than in Wistar rats and the pretreatment of WKY rats with GR 127935 increases midbrain 5-HTP levels [55]. These interesting findings need to be extended to other brain regions and confirmed with more selective agents. However the use of these "anxious" strains of rats promise to be a fruitful model to study the involvement of a subtype of receptor in the development of anxiety and/or other diseases.

Animal models of anxiety

5-HT$_{1B}$ receptors are localized in motor control centers in the brain such as the globus pallidus, substantia nigra and the deep cerebellar nuclei [59].

In general, compounds that decrease 5-HT neurotransmission tend to decrease the level of anxiety, whereas those that increase 5-HT stimulation tend to increase the level of anxiety [25, 60, 61]. Broekkamp et al. [62] have discussed that particuliar animal models are relevant only for the study of one particuliar type of anxiety disorder, and they concluded that the 5-HT$_{1B}$ or 5-HT$_{1D}$ receptors play a role in the "defensive burying" anxiety model and probably mediate antianxiety effects of serotonin uptake inhibitors. Various agonists that exhibit a certain selectivity for 5-HT$_{1B}$ receptors, such as RU

24969, TFMPP and eltoprazine show anxiogenic-like activity in animal models [12] such as the shock probe conflict procedure [63], the social interaction test and the elevated plus-maze test both in rats [64] and in mice [65, 66], although results in conflict tests in rodents are more variable [67]. The rat ultrasonic vocalization (USV) model [68], a putative animal model reflecting anxiety, where USV are elicited by isolating rat pups from their mother and littermates by placing them on a warm (37 °C) or a cold (18 °C) plate has been used to study ligands with different selectivity for various subtypes of serotonin receptors. TFMPP stimulates USV at a low dose at the cold plate and suppresses USV at a high dose under both conditions.

By using more recent compounds it has been shown by Chopin et al. [69] that 5-HT$_{1B}$ receptors might be implicated in anxiety. GR 127935 and SB 224289 (see above) increase the amount of time spent in the light chamber in the two-compartment paradigm in mice, suggesting the drugs to exert anxiolytic-like activity in this anxiety model. The benzodiazepine receptor antagonist flumazenil antagonizes the anxiolytic-like effects of diazepam and of GR 127935. The anxiolytic-like effects of both diazepam and GR 127935 are also inhibited by the 5-HT$_{1B}$ receptor agonist GR 46611 which is inactive when given alone. A combination of an inactive dose of diazepam with an inactive dose of GR 127935 increases the time spent in the light compartment, suggesting a potentiation of anxiolytic effects between these two compounds. These findings suggest that complex interactions can occur between benzodiazepine and 5-HT$_{1B}$ receptors in the regulation of anxiety states as already evoked by Rex et al. [41] concerning 5-HT release and the anxiolytic action of benzodiazepines. Frances et al. [70] have shown that 7 days of isolation induce in mice a social behavioral deficit (decrease in escape attempts) reversed by TFMPP acting through activation of 5-HT$_{1B}$ receptors. The benzodiazepines impair TFMPP-induced increase in escape attempts at behaviorally inactive doses, suggesting that these drugs interact with the 5-HT$_{1B}$ receptors. Therefore again these results add to the knowledge of relations between benzodiazepines and serotonin by specifying the involvement of 5-HT$_{1B}$ receptors. Whether there are similar or separate neuronal substrates modulating serotonergic system and drugs on the one hand and benzodiazepine action on the other hand is an open question and the precise molecular basis by which such interactions may occur requires further study.

By using a murine genetic model, Clément et al. [71] have studied variations in the density of 5-HT$_{1B}$ receptor subtype measured in the brains of parental strains and two other genetically modified populations by quantitative autoradiography with modifications of anxiety-related behaviors. The results have shown that chromosomal fragments, previously shown to be involved in anxiogenic processes, are mainly associated with a variation in the density of the 5-HT$_{1B}$ receptors.

5-HT$_{1B}$ knockout mice

5-HT$_{1B}$ "knockout" mice have been produced by specific ablation of the 5-HT$_{1B}$ receptor gene by homologous recombination [72]. Although these animals, which lack the 5-HT$_{1B}$ receptor, may undergo adaptation during and after development, they represent an interesting model for studying the function of the 5-HT$_{1B}$ receptor and therefore can be used as a pharmacological tool (see the review by Stark and Hen [73]).

Ramboz et al. [74] have found that there is no difference in the level of anxiety between mutant and wild-type mice as judged by their activity in the light/dark model. In contrast, there is a decrease of anxiety state in the 5-HT$_{1B}$ knockout mice compared to wild-type mice in the open-field [75], the ultrasound vocalizations [76], the burying behavior (personal communication) and no difference or a decrease in anxiety in the elevated plus maze [76].

Clinical implications

Sumatriptan is the first compound relatively selective for 5-HT$_{1B/D}$ receptors to be widely used clinically (for the symptomatic treatment of migraine attacks). Other 5-HT$_{1B/D}$ agonists with similar pharmacological properties have recently become available for this indication [77]. Investigations into the possible role of 5-HT$_{1B/D}$ receptors in psychiatric disorders in man have profited from the availability of sumatriptan. Although sumatriptan only penetrates the blood brain barrier to a limited extent, it has proved to be a useful clinical research tool especially for neuroendocrine [78] and behavioral challenge studies.

Although sumatriptan increases plasma prolactin [79], the most specific neuroendocrine response induced in humans by the administration of sumatriptan is a major (greater than five-fold) increase in plasma levels of growth hormone [79]. This effect, which is prevented by prior administration of the non-selective 5-HT$_1$ receptor antagonist, cyproheptadine [79], has been suggested to result from an inhibition of the release of somatostatin *via* stimulation of 5-HT$_{1B}$ heteroreceptors [80].

Obsessive compulsive disorder (OCD) is a psychiatric disorder which is a part of anxiety disorder according to DMS IV. Serotonergic pathways may be involved in the pathophysiology of OCD because selective serotonin reuptake inhibitors are useful in therapy [81, 82]. In addition, in some studies the acute administration of the non-selective 5-HT receptor agonist, m-chlorophenylpiperazine (mCPP) as a probe to study OCD, produces an acute symptomatic worsening in untreated OCD patients [83] that normalizes in patients successfully treated with clomipramine [84, 85]. The two challenges, mCPP and sumatriptan [86], associated with an exacerbation of obsessive-compulsive symptoms, appear to be related to 5-HT$_{1D}$ receptors and it has been suggested that 5-HT$_{1B/D}$ receptors may be supersensitive in OCD [84, 85]. In addition functional imaging with studies of brain single photon emission computed tomography combined with symptom provocation with suma-triptan further supports the role of the 5-HT$_{1D}$ receptor [87, 88]. Since OCD symptoms are unaltered by modification of synaptic 5-HT levels, through tryptophan loading [89] or depletion [90], the receptors involved appear not to be 5-HT release-controlling autoreceptors but more probably 5-HT$_{1B/D}$ heteroreceptors.

Conclusion

In spite of the lack of selective ligands, especially antagonists, available pharmacological data suggest the probable involvement of 5-HT$_{1B/D}$ receptors in the control of a certain number of behavioral activities [12] in general including anxiety states.

Increased levels of anxiety appear to be associated with increased serotonergic activity [61]. The frequent co-existence of high levels of anxiety with depression, often considered to be a hyposerotonergic state is, therefore, somewhat of a paradox. Interestingly, rats exposed to repeated inescapable shocks, such as the "learned helpless rats" not only show a number of "depressive" signs [91], but also exhibit behavior associated with high levels of anxiety [92, 93]. Increased sensitivity of both 5-HT$_{1B}$ autoreceptors and 5-HT$_{1B}$ heteroreceptors could explain this paradoxical situation. More effective feedback regulation (through supersensitive autoreceptors) would result in lower levels of 5-HT release, while up-regulated 5-HT hetero-receptors (on GABA terminals for example) could lead to increased anxiety [12].

By associating behavioral studies of stress and anxiety state with neuro-chemical changes of 5-HT made possible by, for example, the microdialysis experiments, it will be possible with the availability of new selective drugs to identify exactly the target implicated. This sort of approach is quite interesting and merits development in animals in order to be extrapolated to a human state of anxiety. This could elucidate what happens in humans.

At this time it is too early to determine precisely the therapeutic potential of 5-HT-moduline, however the range of therapeutic interest in this endogenous peptide is wide, which is not surprising given the large involvement of the 5-HT system in pathophysiology and anxiety is one of these potential therapeutic interests [44].

Recent studies in OCD [85] suggest that 5-HT$_{1D}$ receptors (probably heteroreceptors) are supersensitive and that their desensitization through long-term administration of 5-HT reuptake inhibitors is related to a therapeutic improvement. A significant gain in the delay of onset of action and possibly greater efficacy can thus be expected by the use of specific direct acting 5-HT$_{1D}$ receptor antagonists in the treatment of OCD.

In conclusion, 5-HT$_{1B/D}$ receptors are clearly involved in a number of basic behavioral activities in animals. Several lines of evidence suggest that changes in the sensitivity of 5-HT$_{1B/D}$ auto- and/or heteroreceptors may be fundamental to psychiatric disorders such as anxiety and OCD. Although it must be admitted that anxiety is a relatively unexplored area for potential new anxiolytics, further investigation into 5-HT$_{1B/D}$ receptor function in psychopathology would appear to be potentially rewarding. In addition the development of new selective compounds, particularly antagonists, will provide therapeutic agents which will be more efficacious and act more rapidly than current medication.

References

1 Baumgarten HG, Göthert M (eds) (1997) *Serotoninergic neurons and 5-HT receptors in the CNS.* Springer-Verlag, Berlin

2 Hartig PR, Hoyer D, Humphrey PPA, Martin GR (1996) Alignment of receptor nomenclature with the human genome: classification of 5-HT$_{1B}$ and 5-HT$_{1D}$ receptor subtypes. *Trends Pharmacol Sci* 17: 103–105

3 Waeber C, Dietl MM, Hoyer D, Palacios JM (1989) 5-HT$_1$ receptors in the vertebrate brain: regional distribution examined by auradiography. *Naunyn-Schmied Arch Pharmacol* 340: 486–494

4 Moret C (1985) Pharmacology of the serotonin autoreceptor. *In*: AR Green (ed.): *Neuropharmacology of serotonin.* Oxford University Press, Oxford, 21–49

5 Engel G, Göthert M, Hoyer D, Schlicker E, Hillenbrand K (1986) Identity of inhibitory presynaptic 5-hydroxytryptamine (5-HT) autoreceptors in the rat brain cortex with 5-HT$_{1B}$ binding sites. *Naunyn-Schmied Arch Pharmacol* 332: 1–7

6 Middlemiss DN (1988) Autoreceptors regulating serotonin release. *In*: E Sanders-Bush (ed.): *The serotonin receptors.* Humana Press, Clifton, 210–224

7 Hoyer D, Middlemiss DN (1989) Species differences in the pharmacology of terminal 5-HT autoreceptors in mammalian brain. *Trends Pharmacol Sci* 10: 130–132

8 Schlicker E, Fink K, Göthert M, Hoyer D, Molderings G, Roschke I, Schoeffter P (1989) The pharmacological properties of the presynaptic serotonin autoreceptor in the pig brain cortex conform to the 5-HT$_{1D}$ receptor subtype. *Naunyn-Schmied Arch Pharmacol* 340: 45–51

9 Starke K, Göthert M, Kilbinger H (1989) Modulation of neurotransmitter release by presynaptic autoreceptors. *Physiol Rev* 69: 864–989

10 Bühlen M, Fink K, Böing C, Göthert M (1996) Evidence for presynaptic location of inhibitory 5-HT$_{1D\beta}$-like autoreceptors in the guinea-pig brain cortex. *Naunyn-Schmied Arch Pharmacol* 353: 281–289

11 Schlicker E, Fink K, Zentner J, Göthert M (1996) Presynaptic inhibitory serotonin autoreceptors in the human hippocampus. *Naunyn-Schmied Arch Pharmacol* 354: 393–396

12 Briley M, Chopin P, Marien M, Moret C (1997) Functional neuropharmacology of compounds acting at 5-HT$_{1B/D}$ receptors. *In*: HG Baumgarten, M Göthert (eds): *Serotoninergic neurons and 5-HT receptors in the CNS.* Springer-Verlag, Berlin, 269–291

13 Moret C, Briley M (1997) 5-HT Autoreceptors in the regulation of 5-HT release from guinea pig raphe nucleus and hypothalamus. *Neuropharmacology* 36: 1713–1723

14 Göthert M, Schlicker E (1997) Regulation of 5-HT release in the CNS by presynaptic 5-HT autoreceptors and by 5-HT heteroreceptors. *In*: HG Baumgarten, M Göthert (eds): *Serotoninergic neurons and 5-HT receptors in the CNS.* Springer-Verlag, Berlin, 307–350

15 Vergé D, Daval G, Marcinkiewicz M, Patey A, El Mestikawy S, Gozlan H, Hamon M (1986) Quantitative autoradiography of multiple 5-HT$_1$ receptor subtypes in the brain of control or 5,7-dihydroxytryptamine-treated rats. *J Neurosci* 6: 3474–3482

16 Offord SJ, Ordway GA, Frazer A (1988) Application of [^{125}I]iodocyanopindolol to measure 5-hydroxytryptamine (1B) receptors in the brain of the rat. *J Pharmacol Exp Ther* 244: 144–153

17 Hoyer D, Clarke DE, Fozard JR, Hartig PR, Martin GR, Mylecharane EJ, Saxena PR, Humphrey PPA (1994) VII. International union of pharmacology classification of receptors for 5-hydroxytryptamine (serotonin). *Pharmcol Rev* 46: 157–203

18 Hartig PR (1997) Molecular biology and transductional characteristics of 5-HT receptors. *In*: HG Baumgarten, M Göthert (eds): *Serotoninergic neurons and 5-HT receptors in the CNS*. Springer-Verlag, Berlin, 175–212

19 Hartig PR, Brancheck TA, Weinshank RL (1992) A subfamily of 5-HT$_{1D}$ receptor genes. *Trends Pharmacol Sci* 13: 152–159

20 Starkey SJ, Skingle M (1994) 5-HT$_{1D}$ as well as 5-HT$_{1A}$ autoreceptors modulate 5-HT release in the guinea-pig dorsal raphe nucleus. *Neuropharmacology* 33: 393–402

21 Davidson C, Stamford JA (1995) Evidence that 5-hydroxytryptamine release in rat dorsal raphe nucleus is controlled by 5-HT$_{1A}$, 5-HT$_{1B}$ and 5-HT$_{1D}$ autoreceptors. *Brit J Pharmacol* 114: 1107–1109

22 El Mansari M, Blier P (1996) Functional characterization of 5-HT$_{1D}$ autoreceptors on the modulation of 5-HT release in guinea-pig mesencephalic raphe, hippocampus and frontal cortex. *Brit J Pharmacol* 118: 681–689

23 Piñeyro G, de Montigny C, Weiss M, Blier P (1996) Autoregulatory properties of dorsal raphe 5-HT neurones: possible role of electronic coupling and 5-HT$_{1D}$ receptors in the rat brain. *Synapse* 22: 54–62

24 Roberts C, Belenguer A, Middlemiss DN, Routledge C (1998) Differential effects of 5-HT$_{1B/1D}$ receptor antagonists in dorsal and median raphe innervated brain regions. *Eur J Pharmacol* 346: 175–180

25 Chopin P, Briley M (1987) Animal models of anxiety: the effect of compounds that modify 5-HT neurotransmission. *Trends Pharmacol Sci* 8: 383–388

26 Glennon RA (1990) Serotonin receptors: clinical implications. *Neurosci Biobehav Rev* 14: 35–47

27 Bolaños-Jiménez F, Manhaes De Castro RM, Seguin L, Cloez-Tayarani I, Monneret V, Drieu K, Fillion G (1995) Effects of stress on the functional properties of pre- and postsynaptic 5-HT$_{1B}$ receptors in the rat brain. *Eur J Pharmacol* 294: 531–540

28 Di Chiara G (1990) *In vivo* brain dialysis of neurotransmitters. *Trends Pharmacol Sci* 11: 116–121

29 Macor JE, Burkhart CA, Heym JH, Ives JL, Lebel LA, Newman ME, Nielsen JA, Rya B (1990) 3-(1,2,5,6-Tetrahydropyrid-4-yl)pyrrolo<3,2-b>pyrid-5-one: a potent and selective serotonin (5-HT$_{1B}$) agonist and rotationally restricted phenolic analogue of 5-methoxy-3-(1,2,5,6-tetrahydropyrid-4-yl)indole. *J Med Chem* 33: 2087–2093

30 Hjorth S, Tao R (1991) The putative 5-HT$_{1B}$ receptor agonist CP-93,129 suppresses rat hippocampal 5-HT release *in vivo* – Comparison with RU 24969. *Eur J Pharmacol* 209: 249–252

31 Moret C, Briley M (1996) Effects of acute and repeated administration of citalopram on extracellular levels of serotonin in rat brain. *Eur J Pharmacol* 295: 189–197

32 Bühlen M, Brüss M, Bönisch H, Göthert M (1996) Modified ligand binding properties of the naturally occurring PhE-124-Cys variant of the human 5-HT$_{1D\beta}$ receptor. *Naunyn-Schmied Arch Pharmacol* 353 (Suppl): R91

33 Lawrence AJ, Marsden CA (1992) Terminal autoreceptor control of 5-hydroxytryptamine release as measured by *in vivo* microdialysis in the conscious guinea pig. *J Neurochem* 58: 142–146

34 Sleight AJ, Cervenka A, Peroutka SJ (1990) *In vivo* effects of sumatriptan (GR-43175) on extracellular levels of 5-HT in the guinea pig. *Neuropharmacology* 29: 511–513

35 Roberts C, Price GW, Jones BJ (1997) The role of 5-HT$_{1B/1D}$ receptors in the modulation of 5-hydroxytryptamine levels in the frontal cortex of the conscious guinea pig. *Eur J Pharmacol* 326: 23–30

36 Moret C, Briley M (1996) Effects of GR 127935 on terminal 5-HT1D autoreceptors and 5-HT synthesis in guinea pig brain. *Soc Neurosci* 22: 1332

37 Gaster LM, Blaney FE, Davies S, Duckworth DM, Ham P, Jenkins S, Jennings AJ, Joiner GF, King FD, Mulholland KR, Wyman PA, Hagan JJ, Hatcher J, Jones BJ, Middlemiss DN, Price GW, Riley G, Roberts C, Routledge C, Selkirk J, Slade PD (1998) The selective 5-HT$_{1B}$ receptor inverse agonist 1'-methyl-5-[[2'-methyl-4'-(5-methyl-1, 2, 4-oxadiazol-3-yl)biphenyl-4-yl]carbonyl]-2,3,6,7-tetrahydrospiro[furo[2,3-f]indole-3,4'-piperidine] (SB-224289) potently blocks terminal 5-HT autoreceptor function both *in vitro* and *in vivo*. *J Med Chem* 41: 1218–1235

38 Tingley FD, Schmidt AW, Rollema H, Clarke T, Lebel LL, Sprouse JS, Howard HR, Desai K, Schulz DW (1998) CP-291,952, a high affinity 5-HT$_{1D}$ antagonist, enhances 5-HT neurotransmission in guinea pig brain. *Soc Neurosci* 24, 1109

39 Briley M, Moret C (1993) Neurobiological mechanisms involved in antidepressant therapies. *Clin Neuropharmacol* 16: 387–400

40 Rex A, Fink H, Skingle M, Marsden CA (1996) Involvement of 5-HT$_{1D}$ receptors in cortical extra-

cellular 5-HT release in guinea-pigs on exposure to the elevated plus maze. *J Psychopharmacol* 10: 219–224

41 Rex A, Marsden CA, Fink H (1993) Effect of diazepam on cortical 5-HT release and behaviour in the guinea-pig on exposure to the elevated plus maze. *Psychopharmacology* 110: 490–496

42 Pellow S, Chopin P, File SE, Briley M (1985) Validation of open: closed arm entries in an elevated plus-maze as a measure of anxiety in the rat. *J Neurosci Meth* 14: 149–167

43 Barth T, Rex A, Domeney AM, Fink H (1993) Effects of cholecystokinin fragments in three animal models of anxiety. *In*: N Elsner, M Heisenberg (eds): *Gene – brain – behaviour*. Georg Thieme Verlag, Stuttgart, 621–645

44 Sarhan H, Fillion G (1998) The therapeutic potential of 5-HT$_{1B}$ autoreceptors and heteroreceptors and 5-HT-moduline in CNS disorders. *CNS Spectrums* 3: 50–58

45 Kawahara H, Yoshida M, Yokoo H, Nishi M, Tanaka M (1993) Psychological stress increases serotonin release in the rat amygdala and prefrontal cortex assessed by *in vivo* microdialysis. *Neurosci Lett* 162: 81–84

46 Vahabzadeh A, Fillenz M (1994) Comparison of stress-induced changes in noradrenergic and serotonergic neurons in the rat hippocampus using microdialysis. *Eur J Neurosci* 6: 1205–1212

47 Pei Q, Zetterstrom T, Fillenz M (1990) Tail pinch-induced changes in the turnover and release of dopamine and 5-hydroxytryptamine in different brain regions of the rat. *Neuroscience* 35: 133–138

48 Clement HW, Schäfer F, Ruwe C, Gemsa D, Wesemann W (1993) Stress-induced changes of extracellular 5-hydroxyindoleacetic acid concentrations followed in the nucleus raphe dorsalis and the frontal cortex of the rat. *Brain Res* 614: 117–124

49 Seguin L, Seznec JC, Fillion G (1997) The endogenous cerebral tetrapeptide 5-HT-moduline reduces *in vivo* the functional activity of central 5-HT$_{1B}$ receptors in the rat. *Neurosci Res* 27: 277–280

50 Hjorth S, Suchowski CS, Galloway MP (1995) Evidence for 5-HT autoreceptor-mediated, nerve impulse-independent, control of 5-HT synthesis in the rat brain. *Synapse* 19: 170–176

51 Carlsson A, Davis JN, Kehr W, Lindqvist M, Atack CV (1972) Simultaneous measurement of tyrosine and tryptophan hydroxylase activities in brain *in vivo* using an inhibitor of the aromatic amino acid decarboxylase. *Naunyn-Schmied Arch Pharmacol* 275: 153–168

52 Moret C, Briley M (1993) Which 5-HT receptors are involved in the modulation of 5-HT synthesis by the 5-HT uptake blocker, citalopram? *Brit J Pharmacol* 108: 96P

53 Moret C, Briley M (1997) *Ex vivo* inhibitory effect of the 5-HT uptake blocker citalopram on 5-HT synthesis. *J Neural Transm* 104: 147–160

54 Roberts C, Thorn L, Price GW, Middlemiss DN, Jones BJ (1994) Effect of the selective 5-HT$_{1D}$ receptor antagonist, GR 127935, on *in vivo* 5-HT release, synthesis and turnover in the guinea pig frontal cortex. *Brit J Pharmacol* 112: 489P

55 Chaouloff F, Aguerre S, Mormede P (1998) GR 127935 and (+)-WAY 100135 do not affect TFMPP-induced inhibition of 5-HT synthesis in the midbrain and hippocampus of Wistar-Kyoto rats. *Neuropharmacology* 37: 1159–1167

56 Chopin P, Moret C, Briley M (1994) Neuropharmacology of 5-hydroxytryptamine$_{1B/D}$ receptor ligands. *Pharmacol Ther* 62: 385–405

57 Martinez DL, Geyer MA (1997) A 5-HT$_{1B}$ antagonist blocks effects of RU 24969 on locomotor, but not investigatory, activity in rats. *Soc Neurosci* 23: 519

58 Middlemiss DN, Hutson PH (1990) The 5-HT$_{1B}$ receptors. *Ann N Y Acad Sci* 600: 132–148

59 Bruinvels AT, Palacios JM, Hoyer D (1993) Autoradiographic characterisation and localisation of 5-HT$_{1D}$ compared to 5-HT$_{1B}$ binding sites in rat brain. *Naunyn-Schmied Arch Pharmacol* 347: 569–582

60 Briley M, Chopin P (1991) Serotonin in anxiety. Evidence from animal models. *In*: M Sandler, A Coppen, S Harnett (eds): *5-Hydroxytryptamine in psychiatry: a spectrum of ideas*. Oxford University Press, Oxford, 177–197

61 Briley M, Chopin P (1994) Is anxiety associated with a hyper- or hypo-serotonergic state? *In*: T Palomo, T Archer (eds): *Strategies for studying brain disorders*, vol 1: Depression, anxiety and drug abuse disorders. Editorial Complutense, Donoso Cortés, Madrid, 197–209

62 Broekkamp CL, Berendsen HH, Jenck F, Van Delft AM (1989) Animal models for anxiety and response to serotonergic drugs. *Psychopathology* 22 (Suppl 1): 2–12

63 Meert TF, Colpaert FC (1986) The shock probe conflict procedure. A new assay responsive to benzodiazepines, barbiturates and related compounds. *Psychopharmacology* 88: 445–450

64 Pellow S, Johnston AL, File SE (1987) Selective agonists and antagonists for 5-hydroxytryptamine receptor subtypes, and interactions with yohimbine and FG 7142 using the elevated plus-maze test in the rat. *J Pharm Pharmacol* 39: 917–928

65 Benjamin D, Lal H, Meyerson LR (1990) The effects of 5-HT$_{1B}$ characterizing agents in the mouse elevated plus-maze. *Life Sci* 47: 195–203

66 Rodgers RJ, Cole JC, Cobain MR, Daly P, Doran PJ, Eells JR, Wallis P (1992) Anxiogenic-like effects of fluprazine and eltoprazine in the mouse elevated plus-maze: profile comparisons with 8-OH-DPAT, CGS 12066B, TFMPP and mCPP. *Behav Pharmacol* 3: 621–634

67 Deacon R, Gardner CR (1986) Benzodiazepine and 5-HT ligands in a rat conflict test. *Brit J Pharmacol* 88: 330P

68 Olivier B, Molewijk HE, van der Heyden JA, van Oorschot R, Ronken E, Mos J, Miczek KA (1998) Ultrasonic vocalizations in rat pups: effects of serotonergic ligands. *Neurosci Biobehav Rev* 23: 215–227

69 Chopin P, Colpaert FC, Moret C, Marien M (1998) Interactions between 5-HT$_{1B}$ and benzodiazepine receptor ligands in the light/dark box anxiety model in mice. *Soc Neurosci* 24: 601

70 Francès H, Khidichian F, Monier C (1990) Increase in the isolation-induced social behavioral deficit by agonists at 5-HT$_{1A}$ receptors. *Neuropharmacology* 29: 103–107

71 Clément Y, Hossein Kia K, Daval G, Vergé D (1996) An autoradiographic study of serotonergic receptors in a murine genetic model of anxiety-related behaviors. *Brain Res* 709: 229–242

72 Castanon N, Ramboz S, Saudou F, Hen R (1997) Behavioral consequences of 5-HT$_{1B}$ receptor gene deletion. *In*: HG Baumgarten, M Göthert (eds): *Serotoninergic neurons and 5-HT receptors in the CNS*. Springer-Verlag, Berlin, 351–365

73 Stark KL, Hen R (1999) Knockout Corner - 5-HT$_{1B}$ receptor knockout mice: a review. Int.*J Neuropsychopharmacol* 2: 145–150

74 Ramboz S, Saudou F, Aït Amara D, Belzung C, Segu L, Misslin R, Buhot MC, Hen R (1996) 5-HT$_{1B}$ receptor knockout – behavioral consequences. *Behav Brain Res* 73: 305–312

75 Zhuang X, Gross C, Santarelli L, Compan V, Hen R (1999) Altered emotional states in knockout mice lacking the 5-HT-1A or 5-HT-1B receptors. *Neuropsychopharmacology* 21 (2 Suppl): 52S–60S

76 Brunner D, Buhot MC, Hen R, Hofer M (1999) Anxiety, motor activation and maternal-infant interactions in 5-HT$_{1B}$ knockout mice. *Behav Neurosci* 113: 587–601

77 Waeber C (1998) The role of 5-HT$_{1B/1D}$ receptors in the treatment of migraine. *CNS Spectrums* 3: 30–39

78 Whale R, Cowen PJ (1998) Probing the function of 5-HT$_{1B/1D}$ receptors in psychiatric patients. *CNS Spectrums* 3: 40–45

79 Franceschini R, Cataldi A, Garibaldi A, Cianciosi P, Scordamaglia A, Barreca T, Rolandi E (1994) The effects of sumatriptan on pituitary secretion in man. *Neuropharmacology* 33: 235–239

80 Mota A, Bento A, Peñalva A, Pombo M, Dieguez C (1995) Role of the serotonin receptor subtype 5-HT$_{1D}$ on basal and stimulated growth hormone secretion. *J Clin Endocrinol Metab.* 80: 1973–1977

81 Zohar J, Zohar-Kadouch RC, Kindler S (1992) Current concepts in the pharmacological treatment of obsessive-compulsive disorder. *Drugs* 43: 210–218

82 Pigott TA, L'Heureux F, Bernstein SE, Hill JL, Murphy DL (1992) A controlled comparative therapeutic trial of clomipramine and m-chlorophenylpiperazine (mCPP) in patients with obsessive-compulsive disorder. *NCDEU Annual Meeting*. May 26–29; Orlando

83 Zohar J, Mueller EA, Insel TR, Zohar-Kadouch RC, Murphy DL (1987) Serotonin responsivity in obsessive-compulsive disorder. *Arch Gen Psychiat* 44: 946–951

84 Zohar J, Insel TR, Zohar-Kadouch RC, Hill JL, Murphy DL (1988) Serotonergic responsivity in obsessive-compulsive disorder: effects of clomipramine treatment. *Arch Gen Psychiat* 45: 167–172

85 Dolberg OT, Sasson Y, Cohen R, Zohar J (1995) The relevance of behavioral probes in obsessive-compulsive disorder. *Eur J Neuropsychopharmacol* 5: 161–162

86 Zohar J (1996) Is 5-HT$_{1D}$ involved in obsessive-compulsive disorder? *Eur Neuropsychol* 6: 54–55

87 Hendler T, Goshen E, Zwas T, Lustig M, Sasson Y, Zohar J (in press) Brain SPECT in obsessive-compulsive disorder during symptom provocation with sumatriptan. *Eur J Neuropsychopharmacol*

88 Stern L, Zohar J, Cohen R, Sasson Y (1998) Treatment of severe, drug resistant obsessive-compulsive disorder with the 5-HT$_{1D}$ agonist sumatriptan. *Eur J Neuropsychopharmacol* 8: 325–328

89 Charney DS, Goodman WK, Price LH, Woods SW, Rasmussen SA, Heninger GR (1988) Serotonin function in obsessive-compulsive disorder. *Arch Gen Psychiat* 45: 177–185
90 Pigott TA, Murphy DL, Brooks A (1993) Pharmacological probes in OCD: support for selective 5-HT dysregulation. *Presented at the First International Obsessive Compulsive Disorder Congress*, Capri, Italy, 12–13 March
91 Sherman AD, Allers GL, Petty F, Henn FA (1979) A neuropharmacologically relevant animal model of depression. *Neuropharmacology* 18: 891–894
92 Vandijken HH, Mos J, van der Heyden JAM, Tilders FJH (1992) Characterization of stress-induced long-term behavioural changes in rats – Evidence in favor of anxiety. *Physiol Behav* 52: 945–951
93 Vandijken HH, van der Heyden JAM, Mos J, Tilders FJH (1992) Inescapable footshocks induce progressive and long-lasting behavioural changes in male rats. *Physiol Behav* 51: 787–794

Anxiolytics
ed. by M. Briley and D. Nutt
© 2000 Birkhäuser Verlag/Switzerland

Brain 5-HT$_{2C}$ receptors: potential role in anxiety disorders

François Jenck[1], Jean-Luc Moreau[1], Jürgen Wichmann[1], Heinz Stadler[1], James R. Martin[1] and Michael Bös[2]

[1] *ROCHE Pharma Division, Preclinical CNS Research, CH-4070 Basel, Switzerland*
[2] *Boehringer Ingelheim, Virology Research Center, Montreal, Canada*

Introduction

Due to their predominant brain localization [1], 5HT$_{2C}$ receptors offer innovative targets for designing novel psychotropic drugs for the treatment of psychiatric disorders. 5HT$_{2C}$ receptors (formerly termed 5HT$_{1C}$) are members of the 5HT$_2$ receptor family [2–4] which also includes 5HT$_{2A}$ receptors (formerly 5HT$_2$ receptors) and 5HT$_{2B}$ receptors (formerly 5HT$_{2F}$ receptors). This G-protein coupled receptor family activates phospholipase C as a transduction mechanism. 5HT$_2$ receptor subtypes mutually share approximately 80% amino acid sequence homology but have distinct distributions in the body that suggest distinct physiological functions. Whereas 5HT$_{2A}$ receptors are found in the brain and periphery, 5HT$_{2B}$ receptors are mainly located in the periphery and 5HT$_{2C}$ receptors are found only in the central nervous system (CNS), widely distributed throughout various brain regions [5]; in most brain areas binding sites, mRNA and immunolocalization of 5HT$_{2C}$ receptors reveal a similar overall distribution [1, 6] and species differences between rat and human brain distribution are limited [7]. Their dense presence in limbic and cortical regions is consistent with a possible important role in affective disorders such as anxiety and/or depression. Lower density but significant functional coupling is found in the basal ganglia [8] while high 5HT$_{2C}$ receptor density is found in the choroid plexus where its functional role remains to be elucidated. Neurotoxic lesion experiments indicate that 5HT$_{2C}$ receptors are mostly postsynaptic but there is also evidence suggesting possible pre-synaptic localization on 5HT nerve terminals [9].

The gene for the human 5HT$_{2C}$ receptor has been cloned and is localized on chromosome Xq24 [10, 11]. Receptor variants exist in the human population, resulting in the substitution of a serine for a cysteine at position 23 in the extracellular portion of the receptor [11]. The ser23 variant seems to have higher *in vitro* affinity than the cys23 variant indicating a possible association between genetic variation of the 5HT$_{2C}$ receptor and disease or response to treatment.

Evidence has been reported for an interaction between the dopamine D4 and the $5HT_{2C}$ receptor genes on reward dependence traits [12]. Multiple functional studies have provided additional evidence for a role of $5HT_{2C}$ receptors in the antidepressant and/or anxiolytic action of marketed drugs. Established antidepressants, including classical tricyclics, mianserin, trazodone and fluoxetine, were found to display moderate to high affinity for $5HT_{2C}$ receptors and to play a modulatory role on brain $5HT_{2C}$ receptor function [13–15]. The antipsychotic clozapine, which has an atypical action against negative symptoms of schizophrenia, also has high pharmacological activity at $5HT_{2C}$ receptors [16, 17].

Findings also support the hypothesis that dysregulated $5HT_{2C}$ receptors may play a prominent role in the pathogenesis of anxiety/depression disorders. Chronic unpredictable mild stress known to generate anhedonic states in rats was found to facilitate, whereas antidepressant treatments reduced, $5HT_{2C}$ receptor function in the rat [18]. Likewise, increased $5HT_{2C}$ receptor responsiveness occurs upon rearing rats in social isolation [19], suggesting that $5HT_{2C}$ receptor-mediated function may exist in a hypersensitive state in depression and that normalization of this dysregulated state may contribute to antidepressant action.

Remarkably, however, $5HT_{2C}$ receptor regulation seems to deviate from classical receptor regulation by exhibiting downregulation after chronic receptor activation as well as receptor inhibition [4, 20–22], which opens interesting therapeutic possibilities for both agonists and antagonists at $5HT_{2C}$ receptor sites. As a matter of fact, this may also provide an element of explanation for the intriguing observation that both 5HT mimetics (i.e. SSRIs) and 5HT receptor antagonists (i.e. trazodone or mianserin) possess therapeutic effects against depression [23]. Additional innovative perspectives are opened by the existence of inverse agonists at $5HT_{2C}$ receptors [24] and of amide derivatives of brain fatty acids recently found to allosterically modulate $5HT_{2C}$ receptor-mediated responses in oocytes and which may represent a novel mechanism for allosteric regulation of $5HT_{2C}$ receptors in the brain [25]. The recent development of high affinity and selective receptor agonists and antagonists for $5HT_{2C}$ receptors [26–29] has generated interest in the therapeutic potential of selective $5HT_{2C}$ receptor ligands as psychotropic agents.

$5HT_{2C}$ receptor agonists

Ro 60-0175, Org 12962 and Ro 60-0332 (Fig. 1) have been characterized *in vitro* and *in vivo* as full and selective agonists at the $5HT_{2C}$ receptor subtype [26, 30, 31] behaviorally well tolerated in rodents and primates [32, 33]. These compounds belong to separate chemical series but share nanomolar affinity for $5HT_{2C}$ receptor subtypes and selectivity over more than forty other receptor binding sites with established functional relevance (including $5HT_{2A}$ receptors and sites on $GABA_A$ receptor complexes).

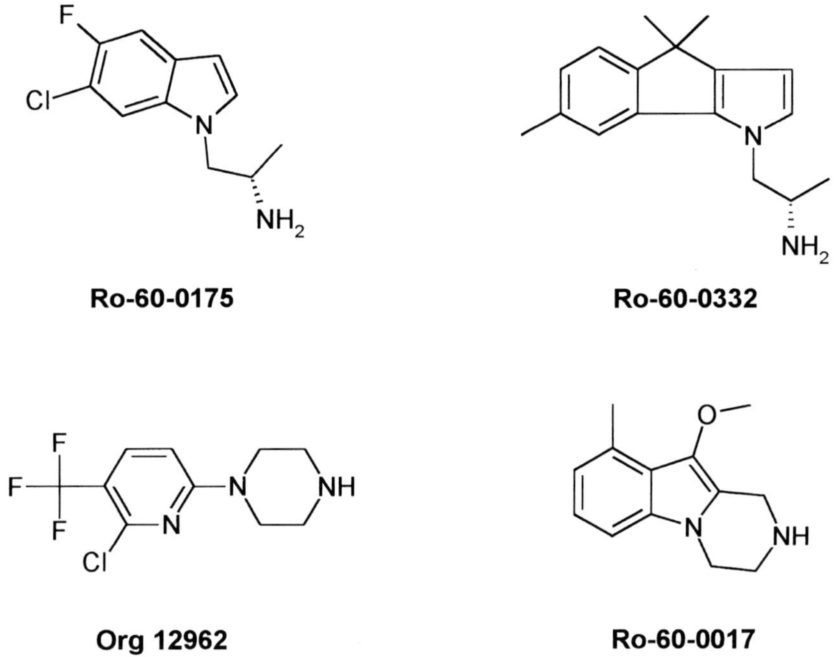

Figure 1. Chemical structures of the selective 5HT$_{2C}$ receptor full agonists Ro 60-0175, Ro 60-0332, Org 12962. Ro 60-0017 is a partial agonist.

Ro 60-0175 and Ro 60-0332 have *in vivo* effects (Fig. 2 and 3) indicative of potential therapeutic action in several animal models of depression [34, 35], panic-like anxiety [35, 36] and compulsive behavior [26, 32, 35]. No effects were observed with selective 5HT$_{2C}$ receptor agonists at non-sedative dosage in standard rat elevated plus-maze and conflict test procedures [32, 35] detecting effects on phobic and conditioned anxiety, respectively.

When active, selective 5HT$_{2C}$ receptor agonists elicited effects with better efficacy than selective serotonin reuptake inhibitors (e.g. fluoxetine). By analogy with the effects of clinically established agents, these results offer a solid argument in favor of potential antidepressant, antipanic and anti-OCD properties for selective 5HT$_{2C}$ receptor agonists. In addition, the fact that Ro 60-0175, Org 12962 and Ro 60-0332 originate from different chemical series but share 1) comparable selective affinity for 5HT$_{2C}$ receptors, 2) a similar agonistic action at those receptor sites in the brain and 3) a common therapeutic potential, further indicates that 5HT$_{2C}$ receptors, in combination or not with other receptor sites, may play an important role in the pathophysiology of affective disorders and thus, in the therapeutic potential of these agonists.

Current thinking on how SSRIs produce their therapeutic effects emphasises the complexity of their action implicating various 5HT receptor subtypes that may be differentially stimulated following facilitated serotonergic trans-

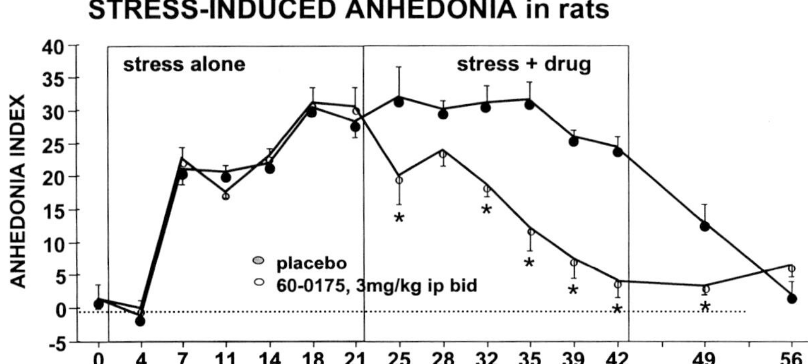

Figure 2. Antidepressant-like effects (top) and antipanic-like effects (bottom) induced by the 5HT$_{2C}$ receptor agonist Ro 60-0175 in rats. Chronic administration of Ro 60-0175 (curative) reverses a chronic stress-induced depressive-like anhedonic state in rats [34]. Fluoxetine, clonazepam and Ro 60-0175 also significantly attenuate panic-like responses in rats [36]. (Reproduced with permission from Jenck et al., *Exp Opin Invest Drugs* 7: 1587–1599, 1998)

mission in the brain [37, 38]. Our data suggest that, among all 5HT receptor subtypes indirectly activated by SSRIs, the 5HT$_{2C}$ receptor may play a major role in the therapeutic properties of SSRIs in the treatment of depression [34, 39], panic anxiety [36], OCD and bulimia [26]. SSRIs seem to have biphasic effects with initial phases of increased anxiety gradually improving into phases of diminished anxiety [40, 41]. While tolerance of those initial signs of anxiety clearly develop, the relative contribution of the numerous receptor types to this adaptation process probably represents a rather elaborate mechanism involving multiple neurotransmitter and neuromodulator systems.

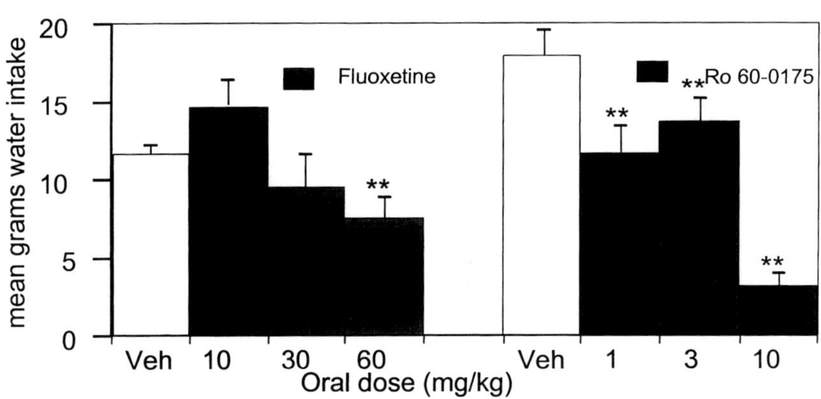

Figure 2. Anticompulsive-like effects induced by the selective 5HT$_{2C}$ receptor agonist Ro 60-0175. Both Ro 60-0175 and fluoxetine significantly reduce schedule-induced polydipsia in rats and displacement behavior such as irrelevant scratching in monkeys [26, 32]. (Reproduced with permission from Jenck et al., *Exp Opin Invest Drugs* 7: 1587–1599, 1998)

Partial agonists at 5HT$_{2C}$ receptors – allosteric modulators

Partial agonists at 5HT$_{2C}$ receptors such as Ro 60-0017 [42] (Fig. 1) may also lead to interesting differentiation in therapeutic potential by preferentially involving specific receptor populations with particular reserves in special regions involved in the control of fear, stress and anxiety. Different receptor isoforms may also accommodate different effects of 5HT$_{2C}$ receptor ligands. Evidence has been reported for the existence of seven distinct isoforms of

$5HT_{2C}$ receptors which are created by mRNA editing (modification of nucleotides) in the second intracellular loop of the $5HT_{2C}$ receptor [43]. This is an important receptor portion for signal transduction and fully edited transcripts show a significant reduction in G-protein coupling leading to a decreased activation of phospholipase C [43]. Editing patterns differ between brain regions, suggesting that differentially edited $5HT_{2C}$ receptors have distinct biological functions in those regions where they are expressed. RNA editing is a new and important mechanism for post-transcriptional regulation of serotonergic signal transduction but criteria by which to judge whether these isoforms are functional *in vivo* remain to be established [44]. In addition to inverse agonism at $5HT_{2C}$ receptors (see below), supplementary innovative perspectives are also opened by the existence of amide derivatives of brain fatty acids found to allosterically modulate $5HT_{2C}$ receptor-mediated responses in oocytes and which may represent a novel mechanism for allosteric regulation of $5HT_{2C}$ receptors in the brain [25].

$5HT_{2C}$ receptor antagonists

$5HT_{2C/2B}$ receptor antagonists such as SB 206553 (Fig. 4) and analogues [29, 45] have been reported to have anxiolytic-like effects in social interaction, elevated plus-maze and conflict anxiety models [46–49], which may suggest a specific action of antagonists in benzodiazepine-sensitive anxiety states.

When tested in our laboratories, comparable effects were observed with some $5HT_{2C}$ receptor antagonists of different chemical classes [28, 45, 50]. However, as confirmed elsewhere [49], none of these antagonists induced effects clearly superior to that of buspirone. Buspirone is itself inferior to standard benzodiazepines such as diazepam or alprazolam in a battery of anxiety tests (elevated plus-maze test, light-dark preference paradigm, stress-induced hyperthermia) sensitive to benzodiazepine and/or non-benzodiazepine receptor ligands in rodents (data summarized in Tab. 1).

Disrupted cross-talk between $5HT_{2C}$ and $GABA_A$ receptors has been proposed to play a role in the anti-anxiety actions of $5HT_2$ receptor antagonists [51]. None of those $5HT_{2C}$ receptor antagonists were found to be active in animal models of depression, panic-like anxiety and OCD (Tab. 1), clearly indicating that different types of fear in animals are differentially responsive to $5HT_{2C}$ receptor manipulations. Certain $5HT_{2C}$ antagonists (i.e. mianserin) possess negative efficacy and are inverse agonists at $5HT_{2C}$ receptor sites.

Inverse agonists at $5HT_{2C}$ receptors

The most exciting developments in the $5HT_{2C}$ receptor field relate to the interesting evidence that constitutively active $5HT_{2C}$ receptors are biologically significant and that certain $5HT_{2C}$ antagonists, such as mianserin, spiperone or

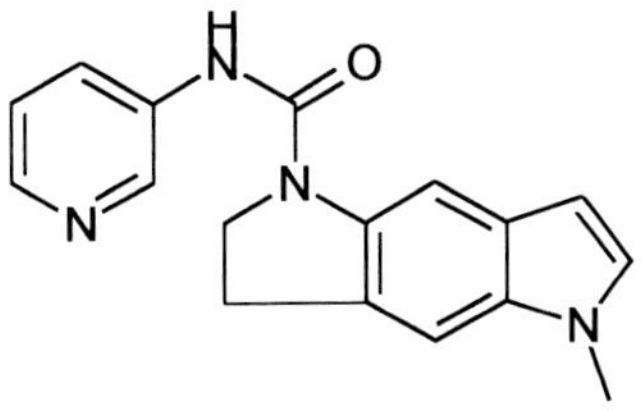

SB 206553

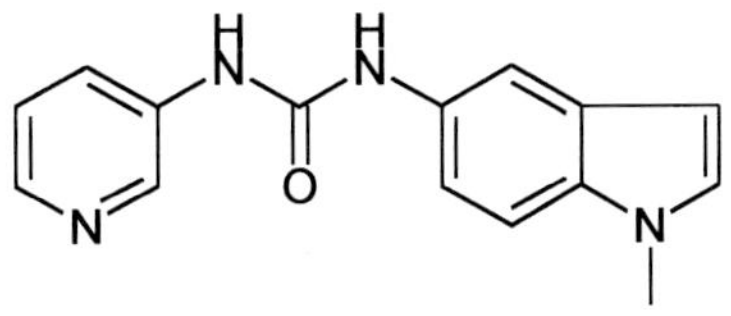

SB 200646A

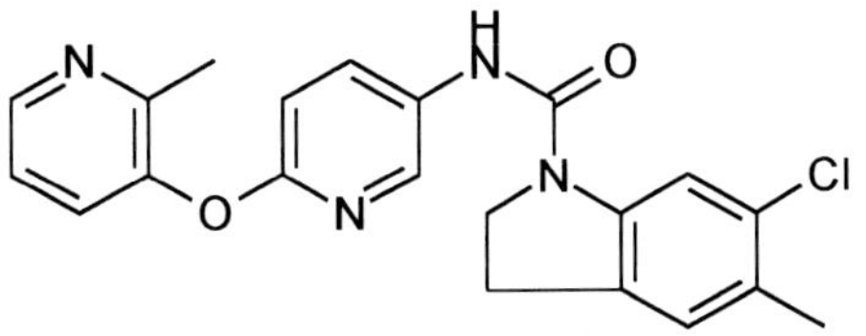

SB 242084

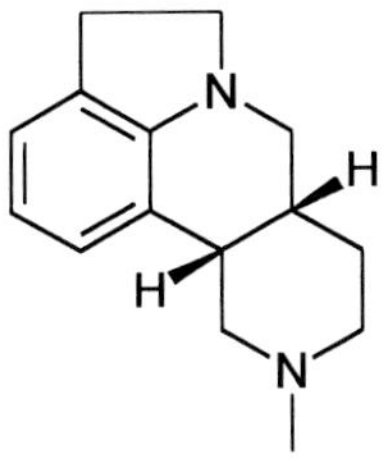

SDZ-SER 082

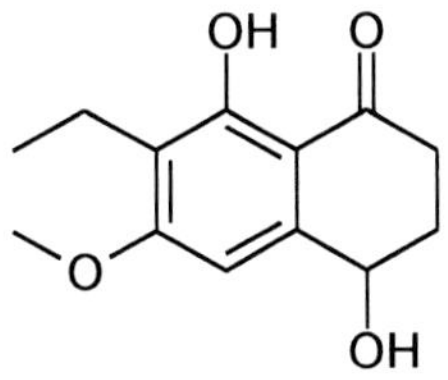

O-Methylasparvenone

Figure 4. Chemical structures of the selective 5HT$_{2C}$ receptor antagonists SB 206553, SB 200646A, SB 242084, SDZ-SER 082 and O-Methylasparvenone.

clozapine, possess negative efficacy at 5HT$_{2C}$ receptor sites [20, 21, 24, 52]. Negative efficacy is a possible and important property of any antagonist at G-protein coupled receptors [53–56]. It depends on a basal level of constitutive, agonist-independent activity that is a likely property of neuronal systems in the living brain and inverse agonists may be of interest when increased constitutive activity results in disease [53, 55, 56]. Recent point mutation experiments show that the 5HT$_{2C}$ receptor can be rendered constitutively active by substitution of serine for lysine at position 312 in the third intracellular loop of the receptor involved in G-protein coupling [57]. This important observation suggests a possible role for somatic mutations in the 5HT$_{2C}$ receptor at codon 312 in the pathophysiology of psychiatric diseases. The S312K mutation at

Table 1. Behavioral profiles of $5HT_{2C}$ receptor agonists and antagonists in a battery of animal models simulating various states on a continuum between anxiety and depression. The value of this classification and its predictive validity are speculative but tend to indicate, when comparison is made to drugs with established clinical activity (BZ, TCA, SSRI), trends for therapeutic potential in specific psychiatric disorders. (Reproduced with permission from Jenck et al., *Exp Opin Invest Drugs* 7: 1587–1599, 1998.)

Animal model	"Etiology"	Cardinal symptom	Reminiscent human disorder	ANX BZ	AD TCA	AD SSRI	$5HT_{2C}$ agonist	$5HT_{2C}$ antagonist
Geller-Seifter, Vogel conditioned fear	chronic conflict	diffuse chronic anx.	GAD	+	0	0	0	(+)
elevated +maze light-dark preference	acute novelty	neophobia	agoraphobia	+	0	0	0	(+)
dPAG aversion	acute brain stimul.	intense acute anx.	panic	+	0	+	+	0
compulsive reactions	acute/chronic discomfort	displacement behaviors	OCD	0	0	+	+	0
behavioral despair tests	acute stress intense	despair	PTSD?	0	+	(+)	(+)	0
chronic mild stress anhedonia	chronic stress mild	anhedonia	depression	0	+	+	+	0

Effects are qualitatively described as + = active, (+) = borderline and 0 = inactive
ANX = anxiolytics
BZ = benzodiazepines
AD = antidepressants
TCA = tricyclics
GAD = generalized anxiety disorders
SSRI = selective serotonin reuptake inhibitors
PTSD = post-traumatic stress disorders
OCD = obsessive/compulsive disorders

least provides a model system for testing agents for inverse agonist activity at constitutively active mutant 5HT$_{2C}$ receptors coupling [57].

The functionally distinct properties of inverse agonists and neutral antagonists following acute or chronic administration may elucidate the mechanisms controlling basal receptor activity states and lead to novel approaches in the development of therapeutic agents [21, 24]. Deramciclane (Fig. 5) is a recent-

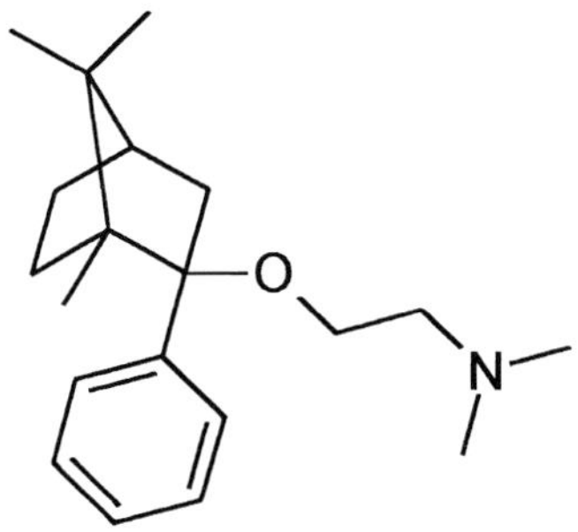

Deramciclane

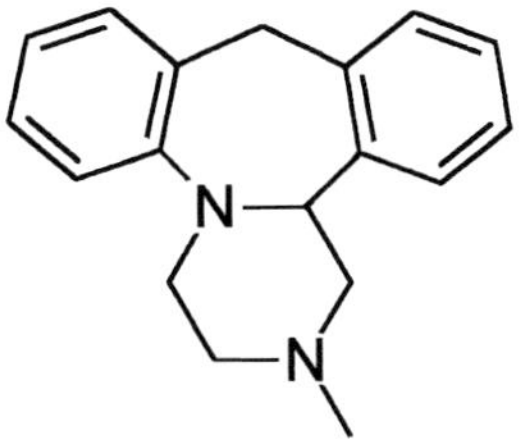

Mianserin

Figure 5. Chemical structures of the selective 5HT$_{2C}$ receptor inverse agonist Deramciclane. Mianserin has also been described with inverse agonistic properties.

ly described putative anxiolytic drug which is a serotonin 5HT$_{2C}$ receptor inverse agonist [58].

The ability of mixed 5HT$_{2A}$/$_{2C}$ receptor antagonists to produce effects on learning and performance has also suggested that they may be acting as inverse agonists at those receptors [59]. The negative efficacy of the "antagonist" ligands mentioned above remains to be elucidated; their effects as inverse agonists or neutral antagonists on different types of fear generated experimentally in animals may lead to interesting differentiation in therapeutic potential. Preliminary differences were observed in our laboratory between antagonists/inverse agonists such as mianserin and presumably neutral antagonists in a model of panic-like anxiety in rats (unpublished results).

Peculiar 5HT$_{2C}$ receptor regulation

Cellular populations of receptors are not static but can be regulated by numerous factors such as cell cycle and physiological or pathological circumstances [56]. 5HT$_{2C}$ receptor regulation seems to deviate from classical receptor regulation by exhibiting downregulation after chronic administration with an agonist as well as with an inverse agonist [4, 21]. Agonists and inverse agonists may elicit conformational changes that probably alter a region of the $5HT_{2C}$ receptor which is important in receptor turnover. Although not fully elucidated, the mechanism by which $5HT_{2C}$ receptors downregulate opens interesting possibilities for repeated administration of both agonists and inverse agonists at $5HT_{2C}$ receptor sites.

Multiple actions at $5HT_{2C}$ sites in the control of fear and anxiety

The opposite patterns of results observed with $5HT_{2C}$ receptor agonists and antagonists in different models are not mutually exclusive but rather suggest that the $5HT_{2C}$ receptor subtype exerts an elaborate control over different types of anxiety: $5HT_{2C}$ neurotransmission selectively modulates specific kinds of anxiety generated by different animal models. This is in line with an interesting theory on the complex action of 5HT on the neural mechanism of anxiety where 5HT is hypothesized and found to either facilitate or inhibit different kinds of fear in different brain regions [60–65]. Different anxiety states in animals or man probably recruit and involve different brain regions and receptor types, either alone or in combination, hence with different symptomatic outcomes. In that respect, the use of non-selective probes such as meta-chlorophenyl-piperazine (m-CPP) are likely to generate contaminated results and cannot be used for elucidation of the physiological machinery involved.

Effects seen with $5HT_{2C}$ receptor agonists are consistent with data on mutated $5HT_{2C}$ receptor-deficient animals suggesting that $5HT_{2C}$ receptors may mediate tonic inhibition of neuronal network excitability [66]. Yet, selective, potent and brain-penetrant antagonists such as SB 242084 do not induce proconvulsant and hyperphagic effects which are characteristic of mutant mice lacking the $5HT_{2C}$ receptor [48, 67, 68]. This stresses the clear biological difference existing between the acute, transient blockade of a receptor with an antagonist and the lifetime absence of a receptor, most probably dynamically compensated by homeostatic counterbalance mechanisms. Predictions of behavioral effects and side-effects of receptor antagonists must therefore be made with caution when based on behavioral phenotypes of receptor knock-out animals.

Functional interactions between $5HT_{2C}$ and $5HT_{1A}$ receptors

It has become apparent that functional interactions exist among 5HT receptor subtypes, as already reported for other receptor systems (i.e. D_1/D_2 interactions). Based on behavioral evidence in animals, specific and reciprocal relationships between $5HT_{2C}$ and $5HT_{1A}$ receptor stimulation have been described [69–72] and a disturbed balance between the functions of these two 5HT receptors has been proposed to contribute to the pathology of depression [73]. Electrophysiological evidence also exists for the presence of $5HT_{1A}$ and $5HT_2$

receptors mediating opposite effects on membrane excitability in the same cell [74]. This is supposed to provide the cell with a flexible mechanism by which serotonin might regulate firing activity. There is also accumulating evidence for functional interactions at the cellular level between G-protein coupled receptors, such as 5HT$_{1A}$ and 5HT$_{2C}$ receptors, that may have an important role in fine-tuning signals from multiple receptor signaling pathways [75]. These physiologically important interactions have been the topic of an interesting pharmacological approach proposing mixed 5HT$_{1A}$ agonists/5HT$_{2C\text{-}2A}$ antagonists as therapeutic agents [76].

Potential advantages of a 5HT$_{2C}$ receptor approach

Selective 5HT$_{2C}$ receptor agonists offer the opportunity to develop new drugs that may have better efficacy and less side-effects than current medications such as SSRIs. SSRIs, which increase the amount of 5HT available for receptor interaction at serotonergic nerve endings, lack the anticholinergic and quinidine-like side-effects of the classical tricyclics [37, 60] but are endowed with a specific pattern of serotonergic side-effects (nausea, emesis, headache, sleep disturbances, initial worsening in anxiety, agitation). Certain subtypes of 5HT receptors have been linked to serotonergic side-effects (5HT$_3$ receptors to nausea and emesis, 5HT$_{2A}$ receptors to agitation and sleep disturbances, 5HT$_{1A}$ and 5HT$_{1D}$ receptors to headache and anxiety, see Fig. 4); 5HT$_{2C}$ recep-

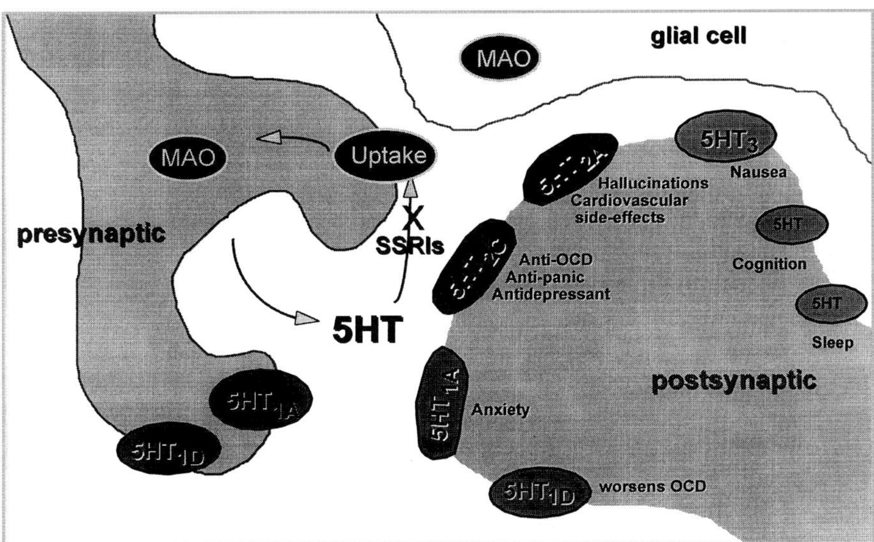

Figure 6. Schematic representation of a serotonergic synapse. For the purpose of clarity, this representation is highly simplified. Without changing the theoretical value of the diagram, presence of all 5HT receptor types on both sides of a single synapse is probably not reflecting the reality. (Reproduced with permission from Jenck et al., *Exp Opin Invest Drugs* 7: 1587–1599, 1998)

tors may be involved in the therapeutic effects of SSRIs, in combination with $5HT_{1A}$ receptors (see below). Their contribution to the effects of hallucinogenic drugs such as LSD has been excluded [77, 78].

Meta-chlorophenylpiperazine (m-CPP), a serotonergic agent that has been used as a neurobiological probe for testing serotonergic function in animals and man, has been found to elicit, under certain circumstances, panic attacks in panic disorder patients [79–81]. While clear evidence exists for anxiogenic effects of m-CPP, disparity in results is considerable as m-CPP challenge tests in patients, healthy volunteers or animals have yielded mixed and inconsistent results. Initial human studies with m-CPP reported biphasic effects on mood, producing positive feelings at low doses and negative feelings at higher doses [82]. Daily administration of m-CPP to healthy volunteers was also found to rapidly attenuate many of its behavioral and physical effects [83] and modest therapeutic effects of chronically administered m-CPP have been reported in some patients [84, 85]. Subsequent studies in animals as well as in man have involved so many variables (route of administration, dosage, purity of chemical samples, animal species and strain, type of patient or volunteer, responder or non-responder, age, experimental paradigm or rating scale) that the numerous discrepancies in the literature on m-CPP's effects and mechanism of action can be viewed as unresolved [86].

In addition, the value of m-CPP as a pharmacologically and clinically meaningful neurobiological probe is highly uncertain. Indeed, m-CPP has a more complex pharmacology than originally considered: in addition to its affinity for $5HT_{2C}$ receptors, it has non-negligible affinity and stimulus effects at $5HT_{1A}$, $5HT_{1D/1B}$, $5HT_{2A}$ and $5HT_3$ receptors [87, 88], is less selective for $5HT_{2C}$ over $5HT_{2A}$ and $5HT_{1A}$ receptor subtypes in man than in rat receptors, may also act as a partial agonist or antagonist at $5HT_2$ sites [89] and also binds to other monoamine receptors such as $\alpha2$ receptors in the human brain [90]. Thus, while predominantly serotonergic, m-CPP is not selective at one receptor subtype, is not a pure agonist, and is not exclusive to 5HT sites; therefore, the anxiogenic effects of m-CPP observed under certain conditions may well result from its interaction with many other non-$5HT_{2C}$ receptor sites. Indeed, anxiogenic effects are also induced by the selective $5HT_{1A}$ receptor agonist flesinoxan in panic patients [91, 92] or by the $5HT_{1D}$ receptor agonist sumatriptan in other types of patients [93, 94]. Finally, m-CPP has pronounced side-effects related to its non-selectivity, which also might induce anxiety as a cognitive side-effect in man [80].

$5HT_{2C}$ receptor antagonists appear to have therapeutic potential in anxiety disorders currently treated with benzodiazepines. Although their efficacy is not that of benzodiazepines in animal models, this class of drug may have an interesting side-effect profile (less sedation, myorelaxation and dependence) and, unlike buspirone, they will need to display a benzodiazepine-like rapid onset of anxiolytic action. Many antagonists with benzodiazepine-like activity such as SB 200646A [46, 47] show mixed affinity for $5HT_{2C}$ and $5HT_{2B}$ receptors. $5HT_{2B}$ receptors are mainly located in the periphery [95] but their controversial presence in the brain and their contribution to CNS effects are unclear. Since 5HT$_{2B}$ receptors are located in the vascular endothelium [96], their detection in many tissues may possibly result from vascular tissue contamination. Although no solid conclusion can yet be drawn on the involvement of 5HT$_{2B}$ receptor-mediated mechanisms in anxiolytic-like effects, it appears that neither 5HT$_{2C}$ nor 5HT$_{2B}$ receptor ligands are adequately competing with benzodiazepine receptor ligands in terms of efficacy in animal models of phobic and conditioned anxiety [49, 97]. Classical tricyclics, mianserin, trazodone and fluoxetine are antidepressants found to display moderate to high affinity for 5HT$_{2C}$ receptors and to have antagonistic properties at brain 5HT$_{2C}$ receptors [13–15]. The antipsychotic clozapine also has significant pharmacological activity at 5HT$_{2C}$ receptors [16, 17]. However, none of these agents is selective at one 5HT receptor subtype and is exclusive to 5HT sites. Therefore, like m-CPP, their value as neurobiological probes is very limited and does not permit to precise examination of the individual pharmacological mechanisms underlying their effects *in vivo*.

Other clinical indications

5HT$_{2C}$ receptor agonists are indicated for clinical development in anxiety and depressive disorders but they may also be efficacious in treating other disorders such as night terrors [98], cocaine addiction [99], eating disorders [100, 101] and in other applications such as irritability, anxious worrying, vulnerability to stress, alcoholism or erectile dysfunction. Activation of 5HT$_{2C}$ receptors is effective in controlling cerebellar glutamatergic transmission and may thereby be useful in the treatment of cerebellar ataxias [102]. Polymorphism at the 5HT$_{2C}$ receptor gene (Cys23Ser) has been proposed for association with a number of psychiatric disorders (i.e. schizophrenia, bipolar disorders, reward dependence, *bulimia nervosa*). Data indicate, however, that the 5HT$_{2C}$ receptor gene does not contribute to the genetic predisposition to migraine and OCD [103, 104] and there is controversy on the association between 5HT$_{2C}$ receptor polymorphism and the response to the antipsychotic drug clozapine [105–107].

Conclusions

Many contradictions about the role of 5HT in anxiety can be explained by the anatomical, pharmacological and functional heterogeneity of 5HT receptor subtypes. Clinical and preclinical data, including those described in this chapter, are compatible with the hypothesis that 5HT has distinct and opposing roles in modulating different kinds of anxiety in different brain regions. 5HT$_{2C}$ receptors are predominantly localized in the brain and their dysregulation may contribute to particular symptoms of anxiety and depression. The marked affinity of several clinically established psychotropic agents' sites (e.g. tricyclic antidepressants, clozapine, fluoxetine) for $5HT_{2C}$ receptor has generated interest in the therapeutic potential of selective, high affinity $5HT_{2C}$ receptor ligands. Like the SSRI fluoxetine, high affinity selective agonists such as Ro 60-0175 and Ro 60-0332 have potent *in vivo* activity in animal models suggestive of therapeutic action against depression, OCD and panic disorders. On the other hand, $5HT_{2C}$ receptor antagonists such as SB-200646A or SB-221284 show signs of anxiolytic-like activity in tests for conditioned and phobic-like anxiety in rodents whereas they are inactive in tests indicative of antidepressant, anti-OCD and antipanic activity. As mentioned earlier, these results are consistent with an important hypothesis proposing that 5HT has a complex, dual action on the neural mechanism of anxiety by either facilitating or inhibiting different kinds of anxiety in different brain regions. They also suggest that $5HT_{2C}$ receptor subtypes play an important role in the therapeutic properties of SSRIs. Certain $5HT_{2C}$ receptor antagonists may possess negative efficacy at $5HT_{2C}$ receptors and, as inverse agonists, may control constitutive receptor activity, possibly characterizing some psychopathological states. Receptor variants exist in the human population and indicate possible associations between somatic mutations in the $5HT_{2C}$ receptor and psychopathology or response to drug treatment. Selective $5HT_{2C}$ receptor ligands may offer innovative and improved therapeutic opportunities for the biological treatment of specific aspects of psychiatric syndromes.

References

1 Molineaux SM, Jessel TM, Axel R, Julius D (1989) The $5HT_{1C}$ receptor is a prominent serotonin receptor subtype in the central nervous system. *Proc Natl Acad Sci USA* 86: 6793–6797
2 Hoyer D, Clarke DE, Fozard JR, Hartig PR, Martin GR, Mylecharane EJ, Saxena PR, Humphrey PP (1994) International union of pharmacology classification of receptors for 5-hydroxytryptamine. *Pharmcol Rev* 46: 157–203
3 Baxter G, Kennett GA, Blaney F, Blackburn T (1995) 5-HT2 receptor subtypes: a family re-united? *Trends Pharmacol Sci* 16: 105–110
4 Roth BL, Willins DL, Kristiansen K, Kroeze WK (1998) 5-hydroxytryptamine 2-family receptors (5-hydroxytryptamine2A, 5-hydroxytryptamine2B, 5-hydroxytryptamine2C): where structure meets function. *Pharmacol Ther* 79: 231–257
5 Pompeiano M, Palacios JM, Mengod G (1994) Distribution of the serotonin 5-HT2 receptor family mRNAs: comparison between $5HT_{2A}$ and $5HT_{2C}$ receptors. *Mol Brain Res* 23: 163–178
6 Mengod G, Nguyen H, Le H, Waeber C, Lübbert H, Palacios JM (1990) The distribution and cellular localization of the serotonin 1C receptor mRNA in the rodent brain examined by *in situ* hybridization histochemistry. Comparison with receptor binding distribution. *Neuroscience* 15: 577–591
7 Abramowski D, Rigo M, Duc D, Hoyer D, Staufenbiel M (1995) Localization of the 5-hydroxytryptamine$_{2C}$ receptor protein in human and rat brain using specific antisera. *Neuropharmacology* 34: 1635–1645
8 Wolf WA, Schutz LJ (1997) The serotonin $5HT_{2C}$ receptor is a prominent serotonin receptor in basal ganglia: evidence from functional studies on serotonin-mediated phosphoinositide hydrolysis. *J Neurochem* 69: 1449–1458
9 Sharma A, Punhani T, Fone KCF (1997) Distribution of the 5-hydroxytryptamine$_{2C}$ receptor protein in adult rat brain and spinal cord determined using a receptor-directed antibody: effect of 5,7-dihydroxytryptamine. *Synapse* 27: 45–56

10 Milatovich A, Hsieh CL, Bonaminio G, Tecott L, Julius D, Francke U (1992) Serotonin receptor 1C gene assigned to X chromosome in human (band q24) and mouse (bands D-F4). *Hum Mol Genet* 9: 681–684

11 Lappalainen J, Zhang L, Dean M, Oz M, Ozaki N, Yu DH, Virkkunen M, Weight F, Linnoila M, Goldman D (1995) Identification, expression, and pharmacology of a Cys23-Ser23 substitution in the human 5-HT$_{2C}$ receptor gene (5HTR$_{2C}$). *Genomics* 27: 274–279

12 Benjamin J, Ebstein RP, Lesch KP (1998) Genes for personality traits: implications for psychopathology. *Int Neuropsychopharmacol* 1: 153–158

13 Jenck F, Moreau JL, Mutel V, Martin JR, Haefely WE (1993) Evidence for a role of 5HT$_{1C}$ receptors in the antiserotonergic properties of some antidepressant drugs. *Eur J Pharmacol* 231: 223–229

14 Akiyoshi J, Isogawa K, Yamada K, Nagayama H, Fujii I (1996) Effects of antidepressants on intracellular Ca^{2+} mobilization in CHO cells transfected with the human 5HT$_{2C}$ receptors. *Biol Psychiat* 39: 1000–1008

15 Pälvimäki EP, Roth BL, Majasuo H, Laakso A, Kuoppamäki M, Syvälahti E, Hietala J (1996) Interactions of selective serotonin reuptake inhibitors with the serotonin 5-HT$_{2C}$ receptor. *Psychopharmacology* 126: 234–240

16 Canton H, Verriele L, Colpaert FC (1990) Binding of typical and atypical antipsychotics to 5-HT$_{1C}$ and 5HT$_2$ sites: clozapine potently interacts with 5HT1C sites. *Eur J Pharmacol* 191: 93–96

17 Kuoppamäki M, Syvälahti E, Hietala J (1993) Clozapine and N-desmethylclozapine are potent 5-HT1C receptor antagonists. *Eur J Pharmacol (Mol Pharmacol Sect)* 245: 179–182

18 Moreau JL, Jenck F, Martin JR, Perrin S, Haefely WE (1993) Effects of repeated mild stress and two antidepressant treatments on the behavioral response to 5HT$_{1C}$ receptor activation in rats. *Psychopharmacology* 110: 140–144

19 Fone KCF, Shalders K, Fox ZD, Arthur R, Marsden CA (1996) Increased 5HT$_{2C}$ receptor responsiveness occurs on rearing rats in social isolation. *Psychopharmacology* 123: 346–352

20 Barker EL, Sanders-Bush E (1993) 5-Hydroxytryptamine 1C receptor density and mRNA levels in choroid plexus epithelial cells after treatment with mianserin and (-)-1-(4-bromo-2,5-dimethoxyphenyl)-2-aminopropane. *Mol Pharmacol* 44: 725–730

21 Barker EL, Westphal RS, Schmidt D, Sanders-Bush E (1994) Constitutively active 5-hydroxytryptamine $_{2C}$ receptors reveal novel inverse agonists activity of receptor ligands. *J Biol Chem* 269: 11687–11690

22 Pranzatelli MR, Murthy JN, Tailor PT (1993) Novel regulation of 5HT$_{1C}$ receptors: down regulation induced both by 5HT1C/2 receptor agonists and antagonists. *Eur J Pharmacol-Molec Pharmacol* 244: 1–5

23 Marek GJ, McDougle CJ, Price LH, Seiden LS (1992) A comparison of trazodone and fluoxetine: implications for a serotonergic mechanism of antidepressant action. *Psychopharmacology* 109: 1–11

24 24Westphal RS, Sanders-Bush E (1994) Reciprocal binding properties of 5-hydroxytryptamine type $_{2C}$ receptor agonists and inverse agonists. *J Pharmacol Exp Ther* 46: 937–942

25 Huidobro-Toro JP, Harris RA (1996) Brain lipids that induce sleep are novel modulators of 5-hydroxytryptamine receptors. *Proc Natl Acad Sci USA* 93: 8078–8082

26 Bös M, Jenck F, Martin JR, Moreau JL, Sleight A, Wichmann J, Widmer U (1997) Novel agonists of 5HT$_{2C}$ receptors. Synthesis and biological evaluation of substituted 2-(indol-1-yl)-1-methylethylamines and 2-(Indeno[1,2-b]pyrrol-1-yl)-1-methylethyl amines. Improved therapeutics for obsessive compulsive disorders. *J Med Chem* 40: 2762–2769

27 Vangveravong S, Kanthasamy A, Lucaites VL, Nelson DL, Nichols DE (1998) Synthesis and serotonin receptor affinities of a series of trans-2-(Indol-3-yl)cyclopropylamine derivatives. *J Med Chem* 41: 4995–5001

28 Bös M, Stadler H, Wichmann J, Jenck F, Martin JR, Moreau JL, Sleight A (1998) Syntheses of O-Methylasparvenone-derived serotonin receptor antagonists. *Helvet Chim Acta* 81: 525–538. 25

29 Forbes IT, Kennett GA, Gadre A et al (1993) N-(1methyl-5-indoyl)-N'(3-pyridyl)ureahydrochloride: the first selective 5HT1C receptor antagonist. *J Med Chem* 36: 1104–1107

30 Millan MJ, Peglion JL, Lavielle G, Perrin S (1997) 5HT$_{2C}$ receptors mediate penile erections in rats: actions of novel and selective agonists and antagonists. *Eur J Pharmacol* 325: 9–12

31 Zhang Y, Dou Y, Ochalski R, Husbands M, Coupet J, Dunlop J (1998) Characterization of the 5HT2C receptor agonist Ro 60-0175 in cells expressing the human 5HT2C receptor. *Soc Neurosci Abstr* 24: 1020

32 Martin JR, Bös M, Jenck F, Moreau JL, Mutel V, Sleight A, Wichmann J, Andrews JS, Berendsen HHG, Broekkamp CLE et al (1998) 5HT$_{2C}$ receptor agonists: pharmacological properties and therapeutic potential. *J Pharmacol Exp Ther* 286: 913–924

33 Millan M, Girardon S, Dekeyne A (1999) 5HT2c receptors are involved in the discriminative stimulus effect of citalopram in rats. *Psychopharmacology* 142: 432–434

34 Moreau JL, Bös M, Jenck F, Martin JR, Mortas P, Wichmann J (1996) 5HT$_{2C}$ receptor agonists exhibit antidepressant-like properties in the anhedonia model of depression in rats. *Eur Neuropsychopharmacol* 6: 169–175

35 Jenck F, Bös M, Wichmann J, Stadler H, Martin JR, Moreau JL (1998) The role of 5HT2C receptors in affective disorders. *Expert Opin Invest Drugs* 7: 1587–1599

36 Jenck F, Moreau JL, Berendsen HHG et al (1998) Antiaversive effects of 5HT$_{2C}$ receptor agonists and fluoxetine in a model of panic-like anxiety in rats. *Eur Neuropsychopharmacol* 8: 161–168

37 Goodwin GM (1996) How do antidepressants affect serotonin receptors? The role of serotonin receptors in the therapeutic and side-effect profile of the SSRIs. *J Clin Psychiat* 57 (suppl 4): 9–13

38 Stanford SC (1996) Prozac: panacea or puzzle? *Trends Pharmacol Sci* 71: 150–154

39 Prisco S, Esposito E (1995) Differential effects of acute and chronic fluoxetine administration on the spontaneous activity of dopaminergic neurons in the ventral tegmental area. *Brit J Pharmacol* 116: 1923–1931

40 Griebel G, Moreau JL, Jenck F, Misslin R, Martin JR (1994) Acute and chronic treatment with 5-HT reuptake inhibitors differentially modulate emotional responses in anxiety models in rodents. *Psychopharmacology* 113: 463–470

41 Allikmets L, Matto V, Harro J (1996) Do the antidepressants have anxiogenic action? *Biol Psychiat* 39: 626

42 Bös M, Jenck F, Martin JR, Moreau JL, Mutel V, Sleight A, Widmer U (1997) Synthesis, pharmacology and therapeutic potential of 10-methoxypyrazino[1,2-a]indoles, partial agonists at the 5HT2C receptor. *Eur J Med Chem* 32: 253–261

43 Burns CM, Chu H, Rueter SM, Hutchinson LK, Canton H, Sanders-Bush E, Emeson RB (1997) Regulation of serotonin-$_{2C}$ receptor G-protein coupling by RNA editing. *Nature* 387: 303–308

44 Martin GR, Eglen RM, Hamblin MW, Hoyer D, Yocca F (1998) The structure and signalling properties of 5HT receptors: an endless diversity? *Trends Pharmacol Sci* 19: 2–4

45 Bromidge SM, Dabbs S, Davies DT, Duckworth DM, Forbes IT, Ham P, Jones GE, King FD, Saunders DV, Starr S et al (1998) Novel and selective 5HT$_{2C}$/$_{2B}$ receptor antagonists as potential anxiolytic agents: synthesis, quantitative structure-activity relationships, and molecular modeling of substituted 1-(3-pyridylcarbamoyl) indolines. *J Med Chem* 41: 1598–1612

46 Kennett GA, Wood MD, Glen A, Forbes I, Gadre A, Blackburn TP (1994) *In vivo* properties of SB 200646A, a 5-HT$_{2C}$/$_{2B}$ receptor antagonist. *Brit J Pharmacol* 111: 797–802

47 Kennett GA, Bailey F, Piper DC, Blackburn TP (1995) Effect of SB 200646A, a 5HT$_{2C}$/5HT$_{2B}$ receptor antagonist in two conflict models of anxiety. *Psychopharmacology* 118: 178–182

48 Kennett GA, Wood MD, Bright F, Trail B, Riley G, Holland V, Avenell KY, Stean T, Upton N, Bromidge S et al (1997) SB 24084, a selective and brain penetrant 5HT$_{2C}$ receptor antagonist. *Neuropharmacology* 36: 609–620

49 Griebel G, Perrault G, Sanger DJ (1997) A comparative study of the effects of selective and non-selective 5HT$_{2C}$ receptor subtype antagonists in rat and mouse models of anxiety. *Neuropharmacology* 36: 793–802

50 Bös M, Canesso R, Inoue-Ohga N, Nakano A, Takehana Y, Sleight A (1997) O-Methyl-asparvenone, a nitrogen-free serotonin antagonist. *Bioorgan Med Chem* 5: 2165–2171

51 Huidobro-Toro JP, Valenzuela CF, Harris RA (1996) Modulation of GABA$_A$ receptor function by G-protein coupled 5HT$_{2C}$ receptors. *Neuropharmacology* 35: 1355–1363

52 Kuoppamäki M, Pälvimäki EP, Syvälahti E, Hietala J (1994) 5HT1C receptor-mediated phospho-inositide hydrolysis in the rat choroid plexus after chronic treatment with clozapine. *Eur J Pharmacol* 255: 91–97

53 Schütz W, Freissmuth M (1992) Reverse intrinsic activity of antagonists on G protein-coupled receptors. *Trends Pharmacol Sci* 13: 376–380

54 Lefkowitz RJ, Cotecchia S, Samana P, Costa T (1993) Constitutive activity of receptors coupled to guanine nucleotide regulatory proteins. *Trends Pharmacol Sci* 14: 303–307

55 Milligan G, Bond RA, Lee M (1995) Inverse agonism: pharmacological curiosity or potential therapeutic strategy? *Trends Pharmacol Sci* 16: 10–13

56 Milligan G, Bond RA (1997) Inverse agonism and the regulation of receptor number. *Trends*

Pharmacol Sci 18: 468–474

57 Herrick-Davis K, Egan C, Teitler M (1997) Activating mutations of the serotonergic 5HT$_{2C}$ receptor. *J Neurochem* 69: 1138–1144

58 Pälvimäki EP, Majasuo H, Kuoppamäki M, Männistö PT, Syvälahti E, Hietala J (1998) Deramciclane, a putative anxiolytic drug, is a serotonin 5HT$_{2C}$ receptor inverse agonist but fails to induce 5HT$_{2C}$ receptor down-regulation. *Psychopharmacology* 136: 99–104

59 Welsh SE, Romano AG, Harvey JA (1998) Effects of serotonin 5HT$_{2A}$/$_{2C}$ antagonists on associative learning in the rabbit. *Psychopharmacology* 137: 157–163

60 Stahl SM (1997) Serotonin: it's possible to have too much of a good thing. *J Clin Psychiat* 58: 520–521

61 Deakin JWF, Graeff FG (1991) 5HT and mechanisms of defence. *J Psychopharmacol* 5: 305–315

62 Beckett SRG, Lawrence AJ, Marsden CA, Marshall PW (1992) Attenuation of chemically induced defence response by 5HT$_1$ receptor agonists administered into the periaqueductal gray. *Psychopharmacology* 108: 110–114

63 Graeff FG, Guimaraes FS, De Andrade TGCS, Deakin JWF (1996) Role of 5HT in stress, anxiety and depression. *Pharmacol Biochem Behav* 54: 129–141

64 Guimaraes FS, MbayAPS, Deakin JFW (1997) Ritanserin facilitates anxiety in a simulated public-speaking paradigm. *J Psychopharmacol* 11: 225–231

65 Mora PO, Ferreira Netto C, Graeff FG (1997) Role of 5HT$_{2A}$ and 5HT$_{2C}$ receptor subtypes in the two types of fear generated by the elevated T-maze. *Pharmacol Biochem Behav* 58: 1051–1057

66 Tecott LH, Sun LM, Akana SF, Strack AM, Lowenstein DH, Dallman MF, Julius D (1995) Eating disorder and epilepsy in mice lacking 5HT$_{2C}$ serotonin receptors. *Nature* 374: 542–546

67 Upton N, Stean T, Middlemiss D, Blackburn T, Kennett G (1998) Studies on the role of 5HT2C and 5HT2B receptors in regulating generalised seizure threshold in rodents. *Eur J Pharmacol* 359: 33–40

68 Nonogaki K, Strack AM, Dallman MF, Tecott LH (1998) Leptin-independent hyperphagia and type 2 diabetes in mice with a mutated serotonin 5HT2C receptor gene. *Nat Med* 4: 1152–1156

69 Darmani NA, Martin BR, Pandey U, Glennon RA (1990) Do functional relationships exist between 5HT$_{1A}$ and 5HT2 receptors? *Pharmacol Biochem Behav* 36: 901–906

70 Berendsen HHG, Broekkamp CLE (1990) Behavioral evidence for functional interactions between 5HT receptor subtypes in rats and mice. *Brit J Pharmacol* 101: 667–673

71 Pomerantz SM, Hepner BC, Wertz JM (1993) 5HT$_{1A}$ and 5HT$_{1C/1D}$ receptor agonists produce reciprocal effects on male sexual behavior of rhesus monkeys. *Eur J Pharmacol* 243: 227–234

72 Maswood S, Andrade M, Caldarola-Pastuszka M, Uphouse L (1996) Protective action of the 5HT $_{2A/2C}$ receptor agonist DOI on 5HT$_{1A}$ receptor-mediated inhibition of lordosis behavior. *Neuropharmacology* 35: 497–501

73 Berendsen HHG (1995) Interactions between 5-hydroxytryptamine receptor subtypes: is a disturbed receptor balance contributing to the symptomatology of depression in humans? *Pharmacol Ther* 66: 17–37

74 Araneda R, Andrade R (1991) 5-hydroxytryptamine$_2$ and 5-hydroxytryptamine$_{1A}$ receptors mediate opposing responses on membrane excitability in rat association cortex. *Neuroscience* 40: 399–412

75 Selbie LA, Hill SJ (1998) G-protein coupled receptor cross-talk: the fine-tuning of multiple receptor-signaling pathways. *Trends Pharmacol Sci* 19: 87–93

76 Millan MJ, Canton H, Lavielle G (1992) Targeting multiple serotonin receptors: mixed 5HT$_{1A}$ agonists/5HT$_{1C/2}$ antagonists as therapeutic agents. *DN&P* 5: 397–406

77 Fiorella D, Rabin RA, Winter JC (1995) The role of the 5HT$_{2A}$ and 5HT$_{2C}$ receptors in the stimulus effects of hallucinogenic drugs. I: antagonist correlation analysis. *Psychopharmacology* 121: 347–356

78 Newton RA, Phipps SL, Flanigan TP, Newberry NR, Carey JE, Kumar C, McDonald B, Chen C, Elliott JM (1996) Characterization of human 5-hydroxytryptamine $_{2A}$ and 5-hydroxytryptamine $_{2C}$ receptors expressed in the human neuroblastoma cell line SH-SY5Y: comparative stimulation by hallucinogenic drugs. *J Neurochem* 67: 2521–2531

79 Charney DS, Woods SW, Goodman WK, Heninger GR (1987) Serotonin function in anxiety. II. Effects of the serotonin agonist mCPP in panic disorder patients and healthy subjects. *Psychopharmacology* 92: 14–24

80 Kahn RS, Asnis GM, Wetzler S, Van Praag HM (1988) Neuroendocrine evidence for serotonin receptor hypersensitivity in panic disorder. *Psychopharmacology* 96: 360–364

81 Klein E, Zohar J, Geraci MF, Murphy DL, Uhde TW (1991) Anxiogenic effects of m-CPP in patients with panic disorder: comparison to caffeine's anxiogenic effects. *Biol Psychiat* 30: 973–984

82 Heninger GR, Charney DS (1985) mCPP, a 5HT$_{1B}$ agonist, produces prolactin, cortisol and growth hormone release and biphasic behavioral changes in healthy human subjects. *Soc Neurosci Abstr* 11: 125

83 Benjamin J, Greenberg BD, Murphy DL (1996) Daily administration of m-chlorophenylpiper azine to healthy human volunteers rapidly attenuates many of its behavioral, hormonal, cardio-vascular and temperature effects. *Psychopharmacology* 127: 140–149

84 Mellow AM, Lawlor BA, Sunderland T, Mueller EA, Molchan SE, Murphy DL (1990) Effects of daily oral m-chlorophenylpiperazine in elderly depressed patients: initial experience with a serotonin agonist. *Biol Psychiat* 28: 588–594

85 Pigott TA, L'Heureux F, Bernstein SE, Hill JL, Murphy DL (1992) A controlled comparative therapeutic trial of clomipramine and m-chlorophenylpiperazine (mCPP) in patients with obsessive-compulsive disorder. *NCDEU Annual Meeting Abstract* 5: 26–29

86 Nutt D, Lawson C (1992) Panic attacks. A neurochemical overview of models and mechanisms. *Brit J Psychiat* 160: 165–178

87 Fiorella D, Helsley S, Rabin RA, Winter JC (1995) 5HT$_{2C}$ receptor-mediated phosphoinositide turnover and the stimulus effects of m-chlorophenylpiperazine. *Psychopharmacology* 122: 237–243

88 Gleason SD, Shannon HE (1998) Meta-chlorophenylpiperazine induced changes in locomotor activity are mediated by 5HT1 as well as 5HT$_{2C}$ receptors in mice. *Eur J Pharmacol* 341: 135–138

89 Thomas DR, Gager TL, Holland V, Brown AM, Wood MD (1996) m-chlorophenyl-piperazine (mCPP) is an antagonist at the cloned human 5HT$_{2B}$ receptor. *Neuroreport* 7: 1457–1460

90 Hamik A, Peroutka SJ (1989) 1-(m-Chlorophenyl)-piperazine (mCPP) interactions with neurotransmitter receptors in the human brain. *Biol Psychiat* 25: 569–575

91 Westenberg HGM, Den Boer JA (1993) New findings in the treatment of panic disorder. *Pharmacopsychiatry* 26: 30–33

92 Van Vliet IM, Westenberg HGM, Den Boer JA (1996) Effects of the 5HT$_{1A}$ receptor agonist flesinoxan in panic disorder. *Psychopharmacology* 127: 174–180

93 Dolberg OT, Sasson Y, Cohen R, Zohar J (1995) The relevance of behavioral probes in obsessive-compulsive disorder. *Eur J Neuropsychopharmacol* 5(3): 161–162

94 Loi V, Lai M, Pisano MR, Del Zompo M (1995) Panicogenic effect of sumatriptan: a pilot study. *Pharmacol Res* 31 (Suppl): 348

95 Wainscott DB, Cohen ML, Schenck KW, Audia JE, Nissen JS, Baez M, Kursar JD, Lucaites VL, Nelson DL (1993) Pharmacological characteristics of the newly cloned rat 5-hydroxytryptamine 2F receptor. *Mol Pharmacol* 43: 419–426

96 Ellis ES, Byrne C, Murphy OE, Tilford NS, Baxter GS (1995) Mediation by 5-hydroxytryptamine$_{2B}$ receptors of endothelium-dependent relaxation in rat jugular vein. *Brit J Pharmacol* 114: 400–404

97 Kennett GA, Bright F, Trail B, Baxter GS, Blackburn TP (1996) Effects of the 5HT$_{2B}$ receptor agonist BW 723C86 on three rat models of anxiety. *Brit J Pharmacol* 117: 1443–1448

98 Wilson SJ, Lillywhite AR, Potokar JP, Nutt DJ (1997) Adult night terrors and paroxetine. *Lancet* 350 (9072): 185

99 Buydens-Branchey L, Branchey M, Fergeson P, Hudson J, McKernin C (1997) The meta-chlorophenylpiperazine challenge test in cocaine addicts: hormonal and psychological responses. *Biol Psychiat* 41: 1071–1086

100 Cowen PJ, Clifford EM, Wiliams C, Walsh AES, Fairburn CG (1995) Why is dieting so difficult? *Nature* 376: 567

101 Dourish CT, Vickers SP, Clifton PG (1998) The selective 5HT2C receptor agonist Ro 60-0175 decreases meal size and accelerates the onset of the behavioral satiety sequence in the rat. *Soc Neurosci Abstr* 24: 1020

102 Marcoli M, Maura G, Tortarolo M, Raiteri M (1998) Trazodone is a potent agonist at 5HT$_{2C}$ receptors mediating inhibition of the N-methyl-D-aspartate/nitric oxide/cyclic GMP pathway in rat cerebellum. *J Pharmacol Exp Ther* 285: 983–986

103 Burnet PW, Harrison PJ, Goodwin GM, Battersby S, Ogilvie AD, Olesen J, Russell MB (1997) Allelic variation in the serotonin 5HT$_{2C}$ receptor gene and migraine. *Neuroreport* 8: 2651–2653

104 Cavallini MC, Di Bella D, Pasquale L, Henin M, Bellodi L (1998) 5HT2C CYS/SER 23 polymorphism is not associated with obsessive-compulsive disorder. *Psychiat Res* 77: 97–104

105 Sodhi MS, Arranz MJ, Curtis D, Ball DM, Sham P, Roberts GW, Price J, Collier DA, Kerwin RW (1995) Association between clozapine response and allelic variation in the 5HT$_{2C}$ receptor gene. *Neuroreport* 7: 169–172
106 Malhotra AK, Goldman D, Ozaki N, Rooney W, Clifton A, Buchanan RW, Breier A, Pickar D (1996) Clozapine response and the 5HT$_{2C}$ Cys23Ser polymorphism. *Neuroreport* 7: 2100–2102
107 Rietschel M, Naber D, Fimmers R, Moller HJ, Propping P, Nothen MM (1997) Efficacy and side-effects of clozapine not associated with variation in the 5HT$_{2C}$ receptor. *Neuroreport* 8: 1999–2003

Anxiolytics
ed. by M. Briley and D. Nutt
© 2000 Birkhäuser Verlag/Switzerland

Glutamate receptor ligands

Phil Skolnick

Neuroscience Discovery, Lilly Research Laboratories, Lilly Corporate Center, Drop Code 0510, Indianapolis, IN 46285, USA

A brief overview of NMDA receptor biology

During the past decade, pharmacological, electrophysiological, and molecular biological studies have yielded a detailed, albeit imperfect picture of the assembly and operation of NMDA receptors in the central nervous system. While a review of all aspects of NMDA receptor biology is clearly beyond the scope of this chapter, it is important to review, however briefly, the salient features of NMDA receptors of particular relevance to drug design and development.

NMDA receptors are broadly and unevenly distributed throughout the mammalian central nervous system (reviewed in [3]). There are eight potential variants of the NMDAR-1 subunit formed by alternative splicing [4, reviewed in 5], and four NR-2 subunits (termed 2A-2D) that arise from distinct gene products [6, 7] reviewed in [3]. *In situ* hybridization studies indicate mRNAs encoding the NMDAR-1, 2A, and 2B subunits are particularly abundant in areas that have been implicated in anxiety such as the hippocampus, amygdala, and cortex [8–10].

Like other ligand-gated ion channels, native NMDA receptors appear to be constituted as hetero-oligomers. While the subunit stoichiometry of NMDA receptors has not yet been evinced, the majority of native receptors are assembled from one or more NMDAR-1 (the murine homologue is referred to as ξ [6]) and one or more NMDAR-2 (the murine homologue is referred to as ε [6]) subunits [11, 12]. Based on neurochemical and electrophysiological studies, NMDA receptors are, at a minimum assembled as tetramers [13, 12]. Further, a subpopulation of receptors is heterogeneous with respect to NMDAR-2 (that is, containing both the NMDAR-2A and –2B subunits), although the proportion of this receptor subtype(s) compared to the total pool of NMDA receptors remains controversial [11, 12, 14].

This hetero-oligomeric structure endows NMDA receptors with multiple interacting "sites" which represent attractive targets for drug development. The ability of ligands to affect NMDA receptor function at these "sites" is determined by subunit composition. Of course, this principle holds for transmitters (i.e. glutamate and glycine) and modulators (e.g. endogenous polyamines such as spermine) [15, 16] as well as for drug candidates. There are examples of subtype selective ligands, as exemplified by the selectivity of ifenprodil for receptors (both native and recombinant) containing a NMDAR-2B subunit [17]. Certainly, the development of subtype selective ligands represents one approach to develop clinical candidates with an acceptable side-effect profile [18, 19]. Nonetheless, direct extrapolation from studies exploring subtype selectivity among binary recombinant NMDA receptors (e.g. NMDAR-1+NMDAR-2A *versus* NMDAR-1+NMDAR-2B) may be misleading, because ligand affinities in receptors that are heterogeneous with respect to NMDAR-2 can differ markedly from the values obtained in receptors assembled with only one type of NMDAR-2 [20]. The co-agonist requirement (i.e. occupation of both a glutamate and a strychnine-insensitive glycine site) [21] for operation of NMDA receptor-coupled cation channels is unique, and has offered a particularly attractive target for pharmacological intervention. Following the demonstration that dizocilpine acts a potent, specific uncompetitive NMDA antagonist [2], compounds which reduce transmission at NMDA receptors at a number of distinct but interacting loci on this family of ligand-gated ion channels have been shown to mimic the effects of clinically effective anxiolytics in one or more preclinical models as outlined in the next section.

Functional NMDA antagonists are active in preclinical tests that predict anxiolytic actions

The recognition that the anticonflict actions of MK-801 [1] were related to NMDA receptor blockade [2] prompted studies to determine: 1) if antagonists acting at other loci on NMDA receptors possess anticonflict actions and 2) the activity of NMDA antagonists in a range of preclinical models commonly used to detect antianxiety agents. Among the earliest reports were those of Bennett and coworkers [22, 23] who demonstrated that the prototypic competitive antagonist AP-7 (2-aminophosphonoheptanoic acid) as well as the heterocyclic compounds, CPP and CGS 19755 increased punished responding in a Cook-Davidson conflict model. At the same time, Stephens and coworkers [24, 25] demonstrated that AP-7 increased both punished responding in the four-plate apparatus and the percentage of time and entries into the open arms of an elevated plus maze. Stephens and Andrews [25] noted that despite the positive results with AP-7, a reliable anticonflict action could not be obtained with MK-801 [25]. These authors note the motor behaviors associated with MK-801, and it is this repertoire of behaviors (hyperactivity, followed at higher doses by ataxia and sedation) that may obscure the potential anxiolytic-like actions of MK-801 and related high affinity uncompetitive NMDA antagonists [26]. These potential confounds may also be reflected in the original Clineschmidt [1] study, where efficacy in the thirsty rat conflict [27] is obtained: "...providing the compound is given 2 or more hours before the test." "MK-801 was without anticonflict activity when administered 1 h prior to study" [1]. Nonetheless, memantine, a low affinity uncompetitive NMDA antagonist (that does not produce the behaviors characteristic of MK-801 and other high affinity channel blockers) was reported ineffective in both the elevated plus maze and thirsty rat conflict tests [28]. In the same study, (+)MK-801 was active in the elevated plus maze, albeit with a lower efficacy than diazepam. It is unlikely that the difference between MK-801 and memantine is related to NMDA receptor subtype selectivity (e.g. [29]).

If pharmacokinetic kinetic issues are not considered, then the basis for many of the apparent inconsistencies present in this literature may be related to the use of $GABA_A$ receptor modulators to validate, and in a sense shape, most procedures currently used to detect anxiolytics (reviewed in [30]). Responses to benzodiazepines and related molecules are thus generally quite robust, and may not be remarkably affected by "subtle" modifications in procedure (e.g. the presence and height of a "lip" on the elevated arms of a plus maze). However, procedural (e.g. strain and species; lighting) and equipment (e.g. elevation and dimensions of a plus-maze) differences that do not dramatically alter the effectiveness of a benzodiazepine may obscure the actions of other classes of compounds, including compounds acting at different loci on the same supramolecular complex, and even extend to compounds acting at the same locus. Such differences may explain a study reporting [28] positive effects with a competitive NMDA antagonist but not with a variety of glycine antagonists in the elevated plus-maze. In the same study [28], positive effects were obtained with MK-801 but not with memantine [28].

Several trends have emerged in this arena during the past decade. Perhaps most notable is a shift from the use of uncompetitive inhibitors like MK-801 to compounds acting at other loci on these ligand gated ion channels that were either not identified or fully appreciated at the time these early studies were conducted. This paradigm shift was prompted, at least in part, by reports of higher "therapeutic indices" associated with compounds acting at these other loci. That is, by comparison to MK-801, these agents produce less toxicity – ranging from a minimal disruption of motor function [31] to the absence of vacuolization [32] in preclinical measures. In clinical studies, the characteristic emergence of side-effects associated with high affinity competitive and uncompetitive NMDA antagonists has not been noted in studies with eliprodil and ACPC [18, 33]. Further, greater structural diversity has been achieved in all classes of NMDA antagonists, resulting in the ability to make broader inferences about the pharmacological actions of a class of compounds that is not based on one or two molecules or structural platforms. Many studies have also incorporated direct injection of NMDA antagonists into brain areas associated with anxiety, a strategy that can sometimes obviate behaviors (e.g. ataxia) obscuring an anxiolytic action. Finally NMDA antagonists have now been examined in a wider range of procedures used to detect anxiolytics. The use of a wide range of preclinical tests – involving both punishment and nonpunishment procedures may increase the possibility of detecting anxiolytics that differ from $GABA_A$ receptor modulators such as benzodiazepines (see above).

The demonstration that occupation of strychnine-insensitive glycine sites is required [21] for NMDA receptor operation stimulated studies to determine the effect of modulating these sites in both conflict and nonconflict procedures. Thus, Trullas et al. [34] reported that both the competitive glycine antagonist 7-chlorokynurenic acid and the glycine partial agonist 1-aminocyclopropanecarboxylic acid (ACPC) were active in the elevated plus maze (in mice), albeit with a lower efficacy than chlordiazepoxide. Corbett and Dunn [35] demonstrated that HA-966, a low efficacy glycine partial agonist, was active in the elevated plus-maze, social interaction, and Cook-Davidson conflict tests. While the efficacies of HA-966, CPP, and dizocilpine were lower than diazepam in this conflict procedure, the efficacies of HA-966 and diazepam were comparable in the nonconflict procedures. A subsequent report [36] demonstrated that the effects of HA-966 were stereoselective in each of these procedures, providing compelling evidence that the efficacy is related to a functional antagonism of NMDA receptors. While the efficacy of (+)-HA-966 remained significantly lower than diazepam in the Cook-Davidson procedure, the efficacy of glycinergic ligands in conflict procedures is not uniformly lower than that of benzodiazepines. For example, Kotflinska and Liljequist [37] demonstrated that increases in punished responding in a Vogel test produced by the glycine antagonist L-701-324 were comparable in magnitude to those produced by diazepam. In the same study, these authors reported that doses of L-701-324 that produce robust increases in a Vogel procedure produced smaller increases in plus maze performance than diazepam. Likewise, ACPC produces a robust increase in conflict responding in the Vogel test at doses that do not affect unpunished responding [38]. Not all investigators have reported anxiolytic-like actions with glycine receptor antagonists and partial agonists. For example, Koek and Colpaert [39] were unable to elicit increases in punished responding in pigeons with kynurenic acid, 7-chlorkynurenic acid, or ACPC. In the same procedure, robust effects were observed with the competitive NMDA antagonists CPP and CGS 19755. While it could be argued that species differences may account for this lack of effect, Karcz-Kubicha et al. [28] reported that a number of glycine antagonists (MRZ 2/570, 2/571 and 2/576) were inactive in the elevated plus maze whilst both HA-966 and L-701,324 produced only a modest increase in the % time spent in the open arms. Further, no significant effects of any glycinergic ligand were noted in a Vogel test by these investigators. These differences could be related to methodological differences and the validation of these tests as discussed above, but may also, at least in part, be attributed to differences in ligand selectivity for NMDA receptor subtypes that are not yet fully appreciated. For example, Kehne et al. [31] compared the effects of two glycine antagonists and found that while the *in vitro* profiles of MDL 102,288 and MDL 100458 were quite similar, the former compound exhibited efficacy and a favorable therapeutic index (>25) in reducing rat pup distress calls, while the latter glycine antagonist had a therapeutic index < 1. A number of glycine antagonists and partial agonists have been examined in the distress vocalization procedure, and generally reduce the frequency of calling in a dose-dependent fashion at doses that do not appear to interfere with motor activity [31, 40]. Glycine-site ligands have also been examined in the potentiated startle test, a nonconflict procedure sensitive to both anxiolytic and anxiogenic agents. Glycine antagonists (7-chlorokynurenic acid) and partial agonists (e.g. HA-966 and ACPC) as well as competitive NMDA antagonists reduce potentiated startle in rats [41].

While there are a number of reports questioning the efficacy of parenterally administered glycine site ligands, a different picture emerges when the anxiolytic potential of these compounds is examined after central administration. Based on the observation [42] that injection of the competitive antagonist AP-7 into the dorsal periaqueductal gray (DPAG) resulted in an anxiolytic effect in the elevated plus maze, Graeff and colleagues [43] as well as others [44, 45] have demonstrated that injection of glycine antagonists (e.g. 7-chlorokynerurinc acid) and partial agonists (HA-966) into this region increases both the % entries and % time spent on the open arms of the plus maze. Further, these compounds also raised the threshold of aversive electrical stimulation of the DPAG [43]. Injection of 7-chlorokynurenic acid into the DPAG was also reported to reverse the anxiogenic actions of the $GABA_A$ receptor antagonist pentylenetetrazole [44]. Robust increases in punished responding in a Vogel test were also noted after intrahippocampal administration of AP-7, MK-801 [45] and ACPC [37], while the increase in punished responding produced by the competitive NMDA antagonist CGP 37849 was accompanied by behavioral disruption including ataxia and muscle hypotonia [38]. Increases in punished responding in a Vogel test have also been observed after intracerebroventricular injection of the glycine antagonist 5,7-dichlorokynurenic acid and AP-7 [47] and intra-acumbens administration of MK-801 and AP-7 [48]. *In toto*, these studies support the notion that NMDA receptor inhibition in circumscribed brain areas may result in a "cleaner" effect absent of performance-based side-effects that accompany parenteral administration.

Several years ago, Wiley and Balster [49] summarized the activities of NMDA antagonists in models used to detect antianxiety agents. If this evaluation were based solely on numbers of studies reporting activity *versus* no effect, the weight of evidence in 1992 clearly indicated that in mammals, functional NMDA antagonists mimic the effects of anxiolytics. During the past 7 years, this balance has even more clearly shifted in favor of the hypothesis that this class of compounds exhibits an anxiolytic-like profile. This shift can be attributed, at least in part, to the increased availability of compounds, notably competitive NMDA antagonists (e.g. CGP 37849, CGP 39551) and glycine antagonists (e.g. MDL 102,288 and L-701,324) that are active in both conflict and non-conflict tests. Further, during the past 7 years, there has been a trend towards an increased use of non-operant based models to assess activity. While it could be argued that operant procedures such as the Cook-Davidson and Geller-Seifter models remain the "gold standards" in anxiolytic research, reliance on these procedures may, in some sense, limit the range of potential anxiolytics that can be detected, perhaps yielding an unacceptable rate of false negatives. While the appropriateness of preclinical models for psychiatric disorders will likely continue to engender debate, there are other lines of evidence that support the hypothesis that NMDA antagonists are anxiolytic. For example, injection of the anxiogenic β-carboline DMCM as well as restraint stress activate mesocortical dopamine neurons, thereby elevating DOPAC levels in the medial prefrontal cortex. Anxiolytics like diazepam block these elevations in DOPAC, and both the glycine partial agonist HA-966 and glycine antagonist L-701,324 are as effective as benzodiazepines in this measure [50].

Activation of NMDA receptors is "anxiogenic": preclinical studies

Identification of a neurochemical pathway or mechanism that is perturbed by a psychoactive drug (e.g. inhibition of biogenic amine reuptake by tricyclic antidepressants, blockade of dopamine receptors by neuroleptics) often leads to a hypothesis implicating that pathway in the pathophysiology of the underlying disorder. In parallel with reports describing the "anxiolytic" actions of NMDA antagonists, other studies described the "anxiogenic" effects produced by NMDA receptor activation.

These studies have generally used the same preclinical tests used to detect putative anxiolytic agents, with an effect opposite to that produced by an anxiolytic (e.g. a benzodiazepine) assumed to reflect an "anxiogenic" action. This assumption is consistent with the anxiety-like syndrome produced by so-called benzodiazepine receptor "inverse agonists" (e.g. β-carbolines such as FG 7142 and 3-carboethoxy-β-carboline) [51–53]. Thus, compounds like FG 7142, which mimic the somatic, endocrine and affective symptoms of anxiety in humans [52], produce effects opposite to those of anxiolytics (e.g. an enhancement of shock-induced suppression of drinking [53]). Examples of the "anxiogenic" actions produced by NMDA receptor activation include: a) the effect of nonconvulsant doses of NMDA to *increase* the rate of distress vocalizations in neonatal rats that have been separated from their mothers [40]; b) the ability of NMDA to decrease social interaction in rats [54]. c) an NMDA-evoked decrease in the time spent on the open arms of an elevated plus maze [54]. Each of these actions can also be evoked by β-carbolines such as FG 7142 and 3-carboethoxy-β-carboline (e.g. [55, 56]).

Other findings extend and complement these observations, supporting the hypothesis that activation of NMDA receptors is associated with increased anxiety. Thus, several studies have demonstrated that injection of glycine into the DPAG (a structure implicated in defensive aversive behavior [57]) reduced the number of entries and the percentage of time rats spent on the open arms of the elevated plus maze [58, 45]. These two measures are highly correlated with fear motivated behaviors (such as hyponeophagia and startle response) among inbred strains of mice [59]. These effects of glycine are compatible with data indicating that synaptic concentrations of glycine are not saturating [60–62] despite its high affinity at strychnine-insensitive glycine sites (e.g. an

$EC_{50} < 300$ nM to activate recombinant NMDA receptors composed of NMDAR-1a/2B subunits in the presence of saturating glutamate/NMDA concentrations [17, 63]. The identification of specific glycine transporters [64–66] with an expression roughly parallel to that of NMDA-R1 subunits may be capable of closely regulating synaptic glycine concentrations [67]. The ability of the glycine-mimetic D-serine to produce dose-dependent effects qualitatively similar to that of glycine in the elevated plus maze [58] indicates that the "anxiogenic" properties of glycine cannot simply be attributed to a nonspecific effect. Another compelling observation consistent with the hypothesis that activation of NMDA receptors is anxiogenic comes from the study of Woods et al. [68]. These investigators demonstrated that NMDA is recognized as a discriminative stimulus in pigeons trained to recognize the anxiogenic 3-carboethoxy-β-carboline [51, 56]. In a separate group of pigeons trained to recognize NMDA, 3-carboethoxy-β-carboline was recognized as a discriminative stimulus. These effects were pharmacologically appropriate in that the benzodiazepine antagonist, flumazenil, blocked the ability of the benzodiazepine receptor ligand, but not of NMDA, to act as a cue. These data indicate that the common interoceptive stimuli produced by these compounds may be related to anxiety.

In toto, these studies demonstrate that, like inhibition of GABA$_A$ receptors, NMDA receptor activation elicits behaviors that are the "mirror image" of those produced by anxiolytics. These data, together with the presence of NMDA receptors in brain structures linked to stress and anxiety, are consistent with the hypothesis that a homeostatic balance between GABAergic and glutamatergic transmission (i.e. the principal fast acting inhibitory and excitatory transmitters in the central nervous system) contributes to the development and expression of anxiety [69].

A Group II metabotropic glutamate receptor agonist (LY 354740) exhibits anti-anxiety actions in preclinical models

If NMDA receptor activation contributes to the development and expression of anxiety, then strategies designed to reduce transmission at this family of ligand-gated ion channels to achieve an anxiolytic action need not be restricted to a "classical" blockade at postsynaptic loci. One promising strategy to achieve this objective is directed at inhibiting glutamate release *via* presynaptic, Group II metabotropic glutamate receptors. The metabotropic family of glutamate receptors are coupled to G-proteins, with Group II receptors (that include mGluR2 and mGluR3 receptors) negatively coupled to adenylate cyclase [70]. Converging lines of evidence indicate that use-dependent increases in glutamate concentration *activate* these group II presynaptic metabotropic glutamate receptors which, in turn, rapidly inhibits glutamate release [71, 72] (reviewed in [73]). There are several possible mechanisms that could explain this negative feedback mechanism for controlling the strength of synaptic transmission, including activation of G protein-coupled inward rectifying potassium channels and suppression of voltage gated Ca^{+2} currents (reviewed in [73]). Because activation of these Group II metabotropic receptors appears to occur during periods of elevated synaptic glutamate concentrations, agonists at these receptors would effectively dampen the excessive glutamatergic transmission associated with anxiety without remarkably affecting synaptic glutamate concentrations under resting conditions.

An emerging body of preclinical evidence is consistent with the hypothesis that activation of Group II metabotropic glutamate receptors will produce an anxiolytic action. This evidence is largely based on studies using LY 354740, a potent, highly selective agonist at Group II metabotropic receptors ([74], reviewed in [73]). Thus, this conformationally constrained glutamate analog was as efficacious as diazepam in reducing fear potentiated startle responding in rats [75] and also reduced the enhanced startle responses in rats provoked by withdrawal from chronic nicotine [76]. No effects on either rotarod performance or hexobarbital sleep time were noted at doses 30-fold greater than those which abolished fear potentiated startle. In the elevated plus maze, LY 354740 significantly increased the time mice spent in the open arms [74, 75] while its enantiomer (LY 368563), which does not activate Group II metabotropic receptors, was ineffective.

Several recent studies have examined the effects of LY 354740 in conflict procedures. Klodzinska et al. [77] reported that LY 354740 increased punished responding in the Vogel test at doses as low as 0.5 mg/kg (i.p.), with an efficacy similar to diazepam. In the same study, significant increases in punished crossings were observed in the four plate test in mice, but these effects were achieved at doses (4–8 mg/kg, i.p.) that also reduced motor activity. LY 354740 has also been examined in Cook-Davidson type conflict procedures in both rats and pigeons [78]. In these studies, LY 354740 did not effect benzodiazepine-type increases in punished responding in either species. However, in rats, this compound increased punished responding during time-out periods between scheduled components, and also increased punished responding during a punishment extinction assay. In pigeons, LY 354740 increased punished responding only when shock was not delivered coincident with reinforcement. Thus, while LY 354740 does not resemble a benzodiazepine in a "classical" (operant) conflict paradigm, it does affect certain elements of operant responding. Given the reported efficacy of LY 354740 in a diverse group of other preclinical models, this drug, or one acting by a similar mechanism, could be used to explore the role of glutamatergic pathways in the development and expression of anxiety in humans.

Conclusions

Clearly, side-effect and safety issues are the most formidable barriers to testing the hypothesis that NMDA antagonists are anxiolytic. However, there are strategies (e.g. subtype selective compounds, glycine site ligands, and low affinity uncompetitive channel blockers) that may either circumvent or minimize the psychotomimetic effects associated with administration of NMDA antagonists (reviewed in Parsons et al. [79]). Based on an emerging body of evidence (reviewed in [73]), activation of group II metabotropic glutamate receptors provides an alternative means of dampening glutamatergic tone without the side-effect and safety issues associated with "classical" postsynaptic receptor blockade. Both approaches merit a rigorous clinical evaluation.

Acknowledgments
I thank my colleagues, Drs. Darryle Schoepp, James Monn, and David Leander for providing preprints of their work.

References

1 Clineschmidt B, Williams M, Witoslawski J, Bunting P, Risley A, Totaro J (1982) Restoration of shock-suppressed behavior by treatment with (+)-5-Methyl-10,11-dihydro-5Hdibenzo[a,d]cyclohepten-5,10-imine (MK-801), a substance with potent anticonvulsant, central sympathomimetic, and apparent anxiolytic properties. *Drug Develop Res* 2: 147–163

2 Wong E, Kemp J, Priestley T, Knight A, Woodruff G, Iversen L (1986) The anticonvulsant MK-801 is a potent N-methyl-D-Aspartate antagonist. *Proc Natl Acad Sci USA* 83: 7104–7108

3 Mori H, Mishina M (1995) Structure and function of the NMDA receptor channel. *Neuropharmacology* 34: 1219–1237

4 Nakanishi N, Axel R, Shneider NA (1992) Alternative splicing generates functionally distinct N-methyl-D-aspartate receptors. *Proc Natl Acad Sci USA* 89: 8552–8556

5 Zukin RS, Bennett MVL (1993) Alternatively spliced isoforms of the NMDAR1 receptor subunit. *Trends Neurosci* 18: 306–313

6 Meguro H, Mori H, Araki K, Kushiya E, Kutsuwada T, Yamazaki M, Kumanishi T, Arakawa M, Sakimura K, Mishina M (1992) Functional characterization of a heteromeric NMDA receptor channel expressed from cloned cDNAs. *Nature* 357: 70–74

7 Ikeda K, Nagasawa M, Mori H, Araki K, Sakimura K, Watanabe M, Inoune Y, Mishina M (1992) Cloning and expression of the E4 subunit of the NMDA receptor channnel. *FEBS Lett* 313: 34–38

8 Boyer P-A, Skolnick P, Fossom LH (1998) Chronic administration of imipramine and citalopram alters the expression of NMDA receptor subunit mRNAs in mouse brain. *J Mol Neurosci* 10: 219–233

9 Watanabe M, Inoue Y, Sakimura K, Mishina M (1993) Distinct distributions of five N-methyl-D-aspartate receptor channel subunit mRNAs in the forebrain. *J Comp Neurol* 338: 377–390

10 Monyer H, Burnashev N, Laurie DJ, Sakmann B, Seeburg P (1994) Developmental and regional expression in the rat brain and functional properties of four NMDA receptors. *Neuron* 12: 529–540

11 Sheng M, Cummings J, Roldan LA, Jan YN, Jan LY (1994) Changing subunit composition of heteromeric NMDA receptors during development of rat cortex. *Nature* 368: 144–147

12 Chazot PL, Stephenson FA (1997) Molecular dissection of native mammalian forebrain NMDA receptors containing the NR1 C2 exon: direct demonstration of NMDA receptors comprising NR1, NR2A, and NR2B subunits within the same complex. *J Neurochem* 69: 2138–2144

13 Behe P, Wyllie DJ, Nasser M, Schoepfer D, Colquhoun D (1995) Determination of NMDAR1 subunit copy number in recombinant NMDA receptors. *Proc R Soc Lond B* 262: 205–213

14 Luo J, Wang Y, Yasuda RP, Dunah AW, Wolfe BB (1997) The majority of N-methyl-D-aspartate receptor complexes in adult rat cerebral cortex contain at least three different subunits (NR1/NR2A/NR2B). *Mol Pharmacol* 51: 79–86

15 Williams K, Zappia AM, Pritchett DB, Shen YM, Molinoff PB (1994) Sensitivity of the N-methyl-D-aspartate receptor to polyamines is controlled by NR2 subunits. *Mol Pharmacol* 45:

803–809

16 Zhang L, Zheng X, Paupard MC, Wang AP, Santchi L, Friedman LK, Zukin RS, Bennett MVL (1994) Spermine potentiation of recombinant N-methyl-D-aspartate receptors is affected by subunit composition. *Proc Natl Acad Sci USA* 91: 10883–10887

17 Williams K (1993) Ifenprodil discriminates subtypes of the N-methyl-D-aspartate receptor: selectivity and mechanisms at recombinant heteromeric receptors. *Mol Pharmacol* 44: 851–859

18 Patat A, Molinier P, Hergueta T, Brohier S, Zieleniuk I, Danjou P, Warot D, Puech A (1994) Lack of amnestic, psychotomimetic or impairing effect on psychomotor performance of eliprodil, a new NMDA antagonist. *Int Clin Psychopharmacol* 9: 155–162

19 Butler TW, Blake JF, Bordner J, Butler P, Chenard BL, Collins MA, DeCosta D, Ducat MJ, Eisenhard ME, Menniti FS et al (1998) (3R,4S)-3-[4-(4-fluorophenyl)-4-hyroxypiperidine-1-yl]chroman-4,7-diol: a conformationally restricted analogue of the NR2B subtype-selective NMDA antagonist (1S,2S)-1-(4-hydroxyphenyl)-2-(4-hydroxy-4-phenylpiperidino)-1-propanol. *J Med Chem* 41: 1172–1184

20 Wafford KA, Bain CJ, Le Bourdelles B, Whiting PJ, Kemp JA (1993) Preferential co-assembly of recombinant NMDA receptors composed of three different subunits. *NeuroReport* 4: 1347–1349

21 Kleckner NW, Dingledine R (1988) Requirement for glycine in activation of NMDA-receptors expressed in *Xenopus* oocytes. *Science* 241: 835–837

22 Liebman JM, Bennett DA (1988) Anxiolytic actions of competitve N-methyl-D-aspartate receptor antagonist: A comparison with benzodiazepine modulators and dissociative anesthetics. *In*: E Cavalheiro, J Lehmann, L Turski (eds): *Frontiers in excitatory amino acid research*. Alan Liss, NY, 301–308

23 Bennett D, Amrick C (1986) 2-amino-7-phosphonoheptanoic acid (AP7) produces discriminative stimuli and anticonflict effects similar to diazepam. *Life Sci* 39: 2455–2461

24 Stephens DN, Meldrum BS, Weidmann R, Schneider C, Grützner M (1986) Does the excitatory amino acid receptor antagonist 2-APH exhibit anxiolytic activity? *Psychopharmacology* 90: 166–169

25 Stephens DN, Andrews JS (1988) N-methyl-D-aspartate antagonism in animal models of anxiety. *In*: E Cavalhiero, J Lehmann, L Turski (eds): *Frontiers in excitatory amino acid research*. Alan Liss, NY

26 Xie ZC, Buckner E, Comissaris RL (1995) Anticonflict effect of MK-801 in rats: time course and chronic treatment studies. *Pharmacol Biochem Behav* 51: 635–640

27 Vogel J, Beer B, Clody D (1971) A simple and reliable conflict procedure for testing anti-anxiety agents. *Psychopharmacology* 21: 1–7

28 Karcz-Kubicha M, Jessa M, Nazar M, Plaznik A, Hartmann S, Parsons CG, Danysz W (1997) Anxiolytic activity of glycine B antagonists and partial agonists – no relation to intrinsic activity in the patch clamp. *Neuropharmacology* 36: 1355–1367

29 Monaghan DT, Larsen H (1997) NR1 and NR2 subunit contributions to N-methyl-D-aspartate receptor channel blocker pharmacology. *J Pharmacol Exp Ther* 280: 614–620

30 Rodgers RJ (1997) Animal models of "anxiety": where next? *Behav Pharmacol* 8: 477–496

31 Kehne JE, Baron BM, Harrison BL, McCLoskey TC, Palfreyman MG, Poirot M, Salituro FG, Siegel BW, Slone AL, Van Giersbergen PL et al. (1995) MDL 100,458 and MLD 102,288: two potent and selective glycine receptor antagonists with different functional profiles. *Eur J Pharmacol* 284: 109–118

32 Hargreaves RJ, Rigby M, Smith D, Hill RG (1993) Lack of effect of L-687,414 (+)-cis-4-methyl-HA-966), an NMDA receptor antagonist acting at the glycine site, on cerebral glucose metabolism and cortical neuronal morphology. *Brit J Pharmacol* 110: 36–42

33 Maccecchini ML (1995) Partial agonism and neuroprotection. *In*: J Grotta, LP Miller, AM Buchan (eds): *Ischemic stroke: recent advances in understanding & therapy*. International Business Communications, Southboro, 140–168

34 Trullas R, Jackson B, Skolnick P (1989) 1-Aminocyclopropanecarboxylic acid, a ligand of the strychnine-insensitive glycine binding site exhibits anxiolytic properties. *Pharmacol Biochem Behav* 34: 313–316

35 Corbett R, Dunn R (1991) Effects of HA-966 on conflict, social interaction, and plus maze behaviors. *Drug Develop Res* 24: 201–205

36 Dunn R, Flanagan D, Martin L, Kerman L, Woods A, Camacho F, Wilmot C, Cornfeldt M, Effland R, Wood P, Corbett R (1992) Stereoselective R-(+) enantoimer of HA-966 displays anxyiolytic effects in rodents. *Eur J Pharmacol* 214: 207–214

37 Kotflinska J, Liljequist S (1998) A characterization of the anxiolytic-like actions induced by the novel NMDA/glycine site antagonist, L-701,324. *Psychopharmacology* 135: 175–181

38 Przegalinski E, Tatarcyzn'ska E, Deren'-Wesolek A, Chojnacka-Wo'jcik E (1996) Anticonflict actions of a competitive NMDA receptor antagonist and a partial agonist at strychnine-insensitive glycine receptors. *Pharmacol Biochem Behav* 54: 73–77

39 Koek W, Colpaert FC (1992) N-methyl-D-aspartate antagonism and phencyclidine like activity: behavioral effects of glycine site ligands. *In*: JC Kamenka, EF Domino (eds): *Multiple sigma and PCP receptor ligands: mechanisms for neurmodulation and neuroprotection?* NPP Books, Ann Arbor, 655–671

40 Winslow J, Insel T, Trullas R, Skolnick P (1990) Rat pup isolation calls are reduced by functional antagonists of the NMDA receptor complex. *Eur J Pharmacol* 190: 11–21

41 Anthony EW, Nevins ME (1993) Anxiolytic-like effects of N-methyl-D-aspartate-associated glycine receptor ligands in the rat potentiated startle test. *Eur J Pharmacol* 250: 317–324

42 Guimaraes FS, Carobrez AP, De Aguiar JC, Graeff FG (1991) Anxiolytic effect in the elevated plus-maze of the NMDA receptor antagonist AP-7 microinjected into the dorsal periaqueductal gray. *Psychopharmacology* 103: 91–94

43 Matheus MG, Nogueira RL, Carobrez AP, Graeff FG, Guimaraes FS (1994) Anxiolytic effect of glycine antagonists microinjected into the dorsal periaqueductal gray. *Psychopharmacology* 113: 565–569

44 DeSouza MM, Schenberg LC, de Padua Carobrez A (1998) NMDA-coupled periaqueductal gray glycine receptors modulate anxioselective drug effects on plus-maze performance. *Behav Brain Res* 90: 157–165

45 Teixeira KV, Carobrez AP (1999) Effects of glycine or (+/–)-3-amino-1-hydroxy-2-pyrrolidone microinjections along the rostrocaudal axis of the dorsal periaqueductal gray matter on rats' performance in the elevated plus-maze task. *Behav Neurosci* 113: 196–203

46 Jessa M, Nazar M, Plaznik A (1995) Anxiolytic-like action of intra-hippocampally administered NMDA antagonists in rats. *Pol J Pharmacol* 47: 81–84

47 Plaznik A, Palejko W, Nazar M, Jessa M (1994) Effects of antagonists at the NMDA receptor complex in two models of anxiety. *Eur Neuropsychopharmacol* 4: 503–512

48 Jessa M, Nazar M, Plaznik A (1996) Effects of intra-accumbens blockade of NMDA receptors in two models of anxiety, in rats. *Neurosci Res* 19: 19–25

49 Wiley JL, Balster RL (1992) Preclinical evaluation of N-methyl-D-aspartate antagonists for antianxiety effects: a review. *In*: J-M Kamenka, EF Domino (eds): *Multiple sigma and PCP receptor ligands.* NPP Books, Ann Arbor, 801–810

50 Hutson PH, Burton CL (1997) L-701,324, a glycine/NMDA receptor antagonist, blocks the increase of cortical dopamine metabolism by stress and DMCM. *Eur J Pharmacol* 326: 127–132

51 Ninan P, Insel T, Cohen R, Cook J, Skolnick P, Paul S (1982) Benzodiazepine receptor-mediated experimental "anxiety" in primates. *Science* 218: 1332–1334

52 Dorow R, Horowski R, Paschelke G, Amin M, Braestrup C (1983) Severe anxiety induced by FG 7142, a beta-carboline ligand for benzodiazepine receptors. *Lancet i* 98–99

53 Corda MG, Blake WD, Mendelson WB, Guidotti A, Costa E (1983) b-Carbolines enhance shock-induced suppression of drinking in rats. *Proc Natl Acad Sci USA* 80: 2072–2076

54 Dunn R, Corbett R, Fieldings S (1989) Effect of 5-HT(""-1A"") receptor agonists and NMDA receptor antagonists in the social interaction test and the elevated plus maze. *Eur J Pharmacol* 169: 1–10

55 File S (1982) Animal anxiety and the effects of benzodiazepines. *In*: E Usdin, P Skolnick, J Tallman, D Greenblatt, S Paul (eds): *Pharmacology of benzodiazepines.* McMillan Press, London, 355–363

56 Insel TR, Hill JL, Mayor RB (1986) Rat pup ultrasonic isolation calls: possible mediation by the benzodiazepine receptor complex. *Pharmacol Biochem Behav* 24: 1263–1267

57 Graeff FG (1991) Neurotransmitters in the dorsal periaqueductal grey and animal models of panic anxiety. *In*: M Briley, SE File (eds): *New concepts in anxiety.* MacMillan, London, 288–312

58 Schmitt ML, Coelho W, Lopes-de-Souza AS, Guimaraes FS, Carobrez AP (1995) Anxiogenic-like effect of glycine and D-serine microinjected into dorsal periaqueductal gray matter of rats. *Neurosci Lett* 189: 93–96

59 Trullas R, Skolnick P (1993) Differences in fear motivated behaviors among inbred mouse strains. *Psychopharmacology* 111: 323–331

60 Salt TE (1900) Modulation of th eNMDA receptor mediated responses by glycine and d-serine in

the rat thalamus *in vivo*. *Brain Res* 481: 403–406

61 Rao T, Cler J, Emmet M, Mick S, Iyengar S, Wood P (1990) *Glycine*, glycinamide, and D-serine act as positive modulators of signal tranduction at the N-methyl-D-aspartate (NMDA) receptor *in vivo*: Differential effects on mouse cerebellar cyclic guanosine monophosphate levels. *Neuropharmacology* 29: 1075–1080

62 Thomson AM, Walker VE, Flynn DM (1989) *Glycine* enhances NMDA-receptor mediated synaptic potentials in neurocortical slices. *Nature* 338: 422–424

63 Harvey S, Skolnick P (1999) Polyamine-like actions of aminoglycosides at recombinant N-methyl-D-aspartate receptors. *J Pharmacol Exp Ther* 291: 281–285

64 Zafra F, Aragon C, Gimenez C (1997) Molecular biology of glycinergic neurotransmission. *Mol Neurobiol* 14: 117–142

65 Smith KE, Borden LA, Hartig PR, Branchek T, Weinshank RL (1992) Cloning and expression of a glycine transporter reveal colocalization with NMDA receptors. *Neuron* 8: 927–935

66 Borowsky B, Mezey E, Hoffman BJ (1993) Two glycine transporter variants with distinct localization in the CNS and peripheral tissues are encoded by a common gene. *Neuron* 19: 851–863

67 Bergeron R, Meyer TM, Coyle JT, Greene RW (1998) Modulation of N-methyl-D-aspartate receptor function by glycine transport. *Proc Natl Acad Sci USA* 95: 15730–15734

68 Woods J, France C, Hartman J, Baron S, Cook J (1988) Similarity of the discriminative stimulus effects of N-methyl-D-aspartate and beta-carboline ethyl ester in pigeons. *In*: E Cavalheiro, J Lehmann, L Turski (eds): *Frontiers in excitatory amino acid research*. Alan Liss, NY, 317–323

69 Trullas R, Winslow J, Insel T, Skolnick P (1991) Are glutamatergic pathways involved in the pathophysiology of anxiety. *In*: M Briley, S File (eds): *New concepts in anxiety, Pierre Fabre Monograph Series edn, vol 4*. Macmillan Press, London, 382–394

70 Schoepp DD, Conn PJ (1993) Metabotropic glutamate receptors in brain function and pathology. *Trends Pharmacol Sci* 14: 13–20

71 Battaglia G, Monn JA, Schoepp DD (1997) *In vivo* inhibition of veratridine-evoked release of striatal excitatory amino acids by the group II metabotropic glutamate receptor agonist LY354740 in rats. *Neurosci Lett* 229: 161–164

72 Scanzfani M, Salin PA, Vogt KE, Malenka RC, Nicoll RA (1997) Use-dependent increases in glutamate concentrations activate presynaptic metabotropic glutamate receptors. *Nature* 385: 630–634

73 Schoepp DD, Monn JA, Marek GJ, Aghajanian G, Moghaddam B (1999) LY354740: A systemically active mGlu2/3 receptor agonist. *CNS Drug Rev* 5: 1–12

74 Monn JA, Valli MJ, Massey SM, Wright RA, Salhoff CR, Johnson BG, Howe T, Alt CA, Rhodes GA, Robey RL, Griffey KR, Tizzano JP, Kallman MJ, Helton D R, Schoepp DD (1997) Design, synthesis and pharmacological characterization of (+)-2-Aminobicyclo-[3.1.0.]hexane-2,6-dicarboxylic acid (LY 354740): a potent, selective, and orally active group 2 metabotropic glutamate receptor antagonist possessing anticonvulsant and anxiolytic properties. *J Med Chem* 40: 528–537

75 Helton DR, Tizzano DR, Monn JA, Schoepp DD, Kallman MJ (1998) Anxiolytic and side-effect profile of LY 354740: a potent, highly selective, orally active agonist for Group II metabotropic glutamate receptors. *J Pharmacol Exp Ther* 284: 651–660

76 Helton DR, Tizzano JP, Monn JA, Schoepp DD, Kallman MJ (1997) LY 354740: a metabotropic glutamate receptor agonist which ameliorates symptoms of nicotine withdrawal in rats. *Neuropharmacol* 36: 1511–1516

77 Klodzinska A, Chojnacka-Wojcik E, Palucha A, Branski P, Popik P, Pilc A (1999) Potential anti-anxiety and anti-addictive effects of LY 354740, a selective group II glutamate metabotropic receptor agonist in animal models. *Neuropharmacology* 38: 1831–1839

78 Benvenga MJ, Overshiner CD, Monn JA, Leander JD (1999) Disinhibitory effects of LY354740, a new mGluR2 agonist, on behaviors suppressed by electric shock. *Drug Dev Res* 47: 37–44

79 Parsons CG, Danysz W, Quack G (1998) Glutamate in CNS Disorders as a target for drug development: an update. *Drug News Perspect* 11: 523–569

Anxiolytics
ed. by M. Briley and D. Nutt
© 2000 Birkhäuser Verlag/Switzerland

Peptide receptors as targets for anxiolytic drugs

Spilios V. Argyropoulos and David J. Nutt

Psychopharmacology Unit, School of Medical Sciences, University Walk, Bristol BS8 1TD, UK

The field of neuropeptides has seen great progress in recent years. New peptides have been identified in the brain and the technical advances, such as *in situ* hybridization and antisense probes, have facilitated their study. A number of neuropeptide receptors have been fully or partially characterised, while the development of specific receptor ligands (agonists and antagonists) helps to elucidate their functional role. Most of the research so far has been conducted in animals, but human data have started to accumulate.

Neuropeptides are widespread in the central nervous system but it appears that they are virtually always co-localised with at least one of the classic neurotransmitters. This led to some interesting hypotheses about their role. Neurons, affected by the information they receive, may release a cocktail of transmitters, depending on differential patterns of afferent firing. In turn, this allows for a broad spectrum of potential actions, and differential temporal signalling, faster or slower. Neuropeptides are produced in the ribosomes and their level may vary considerably in different conditions. Generally, once released, they are replaced by new synthesis, with little or no reuptake at synaptic level. They are usually released following small elevation in the Ca concentration in the cytoplasm, while biogenic amine transmitters are released after higher elevations of Ca in the synapses. The neuropeptide receptors cloned so far tend to be coupled with G proteins [1].

Despite the progress in knowledge and the development of exciting hypotheses, no major breakthrough in the neuropeptide clinical psychopharmacology has taken place yet. Anxiety is only one of the areas of psychopathology for which an important functional role for these transmitters and modulators is proposed, and research for potential anxiolytic compounds is well under way. The hope is that they will be devoid of the problems of traditional anxiolytics, such as the benzodiazepines, namely tolerance, dependence, and interaction with alcohol. Ideally, in order to prove useful in clinical practice, the neuropeptide receptor ligands should be potent, have good oral bioavailability, be able to cross the blood-brain barrier and have a reasonably long duration of action [2].

This review will focus mainly on the human research carried out in this field, as well as theoretical prospects and avenues for future research. We will attempt to cover the neuropeptides that have so far been linked with the modulation of anxiety. Review of the vast animal literature in this area is beyond the scope of this chapter. However, some basic findings will be presented and the reader will be directed to relevant sources covering this topic.

Cholecystokinin (CCK)

Cholecystokinin (the "gallbladder mover") was originally discovered in the gut in 1928, by Ivy and Oldberg, where it was shown to regulate pancreatic and bile secretion. Following Pearse's idea [3] that polypeptide-producing endocrine cells originating from the embryonic neural crest are of neuronal origin, it was a matter of time before these peptides were identified in the brain [4]. CCK was the first such peptide to be discovered in the central nervous system [5].

It is currently recognised as the most widely distributed neuropeptide in the brain. It co-exists and interacts extensively with a number of other neurotransmitters and neuromodulators such as dopamine, serotonin, GABA, noradrenaline, excitatory aminoacids, opioid peptides, neuropeptide Y, substance P and vasoactive intestinal peptide. Several active forms of cholecystokinin exist, but the predominant variants in the central nervous system are the sulfated octapeptide (CCK-8s) and, to a lesser extent, the unsulfated tetrapeptide (CCK-4). The CCK pathways in the brain are not completely understood yet. It appears that the peptide is synthetised in the cortex, hippocampus and substantia nigra. High levels are found in caudate nucleus and putamen, with substantial amounts seen in nucleus accumbens, septum, thalamus, periaqueductal grey matter and substantia nigra.

Two different CCK receptors have been recognised. CCK-A binds with both CCK-8s and CCK-4, while CCK-B binds with CCK-4 and its synthetic pentapeptide analogue, pentagastrin. CCK-A receptors are found only in some areas of the brain, such as hypothalamus and nucleus accumbens, but CCK-B receptors are much more widely distributed. High levels appear in the cortex, olfactory bulb, nucleus accumbens, amygdala, hippocampus, cerebellum and hypothalamus. Apart from the postulated involvement of CCK in learning, memory, feeding behaviour, pain perception and schizophrenia, the distribution of this peptide led to speculation about its role in anxiety, and various CCK ligands have been studied extensively in animals and, to a lesser extent, in humans [4, 6].

The animal data of CCK involvement in anxiety are critically reviewed by Griebel [6]. In summary, the studies show that stimulation of CCK receptors is anxiogenic, and this effect is counteracted by CCK receptor antagonists. However, the results are far from consistent. This effect of CCK seems to depend on baseline anxiety levels. Various other transmitters, such as serotonin, dopamine, acetylcholine, opiates, and corticotropin-releasing factor, may participate in this action. Similarly, the results of both CCK-A and CCK-B antagonists in animals are somewhat discrepant. However, as Griebel

[6] recognises, there are considerable methodological shortcomings in the animal models of anxiety used so far. Perhaps new models relevant to CCK need to be developed. In humans the effect of slow infusion of CCK-4 (0.5 mg over 60 min) on the acoustic startle response (ASR) has been studied in healthy volunteers by measuring eye blink response to acoustic stimuli. ASR is a useful model since it is potentiated by anxiety, fear and anxiogenic drugs, and reduced by sedative and anxiolytic drugs. CCK-4 produced an increase of eye blink startle amplitude from baseline. This was in contrast to the decrease recorded with placebo infusion. The subjects receiving CCK-4 reported mild increase in anxiety during the first stage of the infusion, followed by fatigue as the procedure went on. Activation of the hypothalamo-pituitary-adrenal (HPA) axis was also observed, with increases in plasma concentrations of adreno-corticotropic hormone (ACTH) and cortisol. Prolactin and growth hormone (GH) were increased as well. Thus, the effects of CCK may be mediated *via* the stress response of the HPA axis, through an increase of corticotropin-releasing factor (CRF) (see later). CRF is also known to augment the ASR [7].

De Montigny [8] observed in an open study that intravenous bolus injection of CCK-4 induced panic attacks in healthy volunteers. Van Megen et al. [4] review the extensive data from CCK provocation studies in healthy volunteers and anxiety patients. CCK-4 has been convincingly shown to induce panic attacks in panic patients, at a higher rate than carbon dioxide. Compared with the natural panic attacks, the ones elicited with CCK are identical in symptomatology but more abrupt in onset (within a minute from the bolus injection), and have shorter duration. The result is dose related, with 50 µg producing panic in virtually all subjects. While healthy volunteers also panic with CCK-4, panic patients are significantly more susceptible to this effect of the peptide. Studies with pentagastrin have produced similar results [4]. Further, pentagastrin induced panic attacks in patients with obsessive compulsive disorder [9], and generalised anxiety disorder [10], significantly more so than placebo. In a study comparing social phobics and healthy controls, the patients experienced more panic attacks with pentagastrin than the controls, although the result did not reach statistical significance, perhaps due to small sample size (n = 7) in each group [11]. This indicates that cholecystokinin is anxiogenic irrespective of the nosological background of the subjects tested. Whether this effect is due to increased availability of the transmitter *via* enhanced firing of CCK neurons or due to increased receptor sensitivity is still unclear [4].

Javanmard et al. [12] attempted to identify the neuroanatomic correlates of CCK-4 induced panic attacks in healthy volunteers, using positron emission tomography (PET) scanning. In their study design they incorporated a scan during the anticipatory anxiety phase, as well as a second scan at two different time points of the CCK-4 infusion, in an attempt to determine the time effect of a panic attack on brain activity. In one group of volunteers, the second scan was performed during the first minute after the CCK challenge, corresponding to the initiation of the panic attack. In the second group, the scan was performed during the second minute after the infusion of the drug, at the peak expression of the panic symptomatology. During the anticipatory phase, regional cerebral blood flow (rCBF) increased in the left anterior cingulate, left lateral sulcus and left medial and inferior frontal gyri. Decreased rCBF was seen in the left occipital region and right parahippocampal area. The early effect of CCK-4 was an increase in rCBF in the hypothalamic area, more to the left. This increase extended to the brain stem and the cerebellum. The scan at the height of panic anxiety showed a bilaterally increased rCBF in the claustrum and insula, although the change was larger in the left side again. Further, increases were observed in left superior temporal gyrus, right amygdala and cerebellum. Decrease in rCBF in the right medial frontal area was also seen. Thus, the effect of anticipatory anxiety on brain activation appeared to be different from the panic effect produced by CCK-4. Following the challenge, significant increases of ACTH, cortisol, GH and prolactin were measured. Based on the above, the authors proposed a neural circuit involved in panic attacks. The initial proprioceptive sensations, in this case induced by CCK-4, are relayed from thalamus to amygdala and hippocampus, where the information is integrated and assessed. This information also activates the neuroendocrine response *via* the hypothalamus, and it is evaluated in the cortex (claustrum and insula). According to this model, a panic attack is initiated in the brain stem and then spreads in a number of other structures that assess the threat and respond to it. The findings of the above study, and the proposed circuit of panic anxiety are, generally, in keeping with the evidence produced by neuroimaging studies of panic and other anxiety disorders, whether at rest or after a challenge [13]. Although activation studies have revealed the involvement of many brain areas in anxiety, the results depend on the condition and the paradigm used each time. However, the anterior cingulate, the orbitofrontal cortex and the insula are implicated in all the studies conducted so far [14]. Therefore, these structures appear to represent the anatomical substrate of the experience of anxiety, where a variety of sensory stimuli, neurochemical abnormalities and cognitive distortions may converge, or exert their independent effects.

In an open study, the panicogenic effect of CCK-4 in patients with panic disorder was blocked by pre-treatment with imipramine [15]. A similar result was obtained in a double-blind, placebo-controlled study with fluvoxamine [16]. In this study, panic patients were challenged with CCK-4 before and after treatment with either fluvoxamine or placebo. The number of panic attacks elicited by CCK-4 intravenous injection was significantly lower following treatment with fluvoxamine, compared to the number of attacks elicited before treatment. On the contrary, the placebo-treated group did not show a significant difference in the number of panic attacks before and after treatment (Fig. 1). When the panic rate, following CCK-4 infusion, in responders (irrespective of whether they were treated with fluvoxamine or placebo) was compared to the panic rate in non-responders, a significant reduction was observed in the responder group (Fig. 2). The authors concluded that pre-treatment with fluvoxamine, a drug belonging to the serotonin reuptake inhibitor (SSRI)

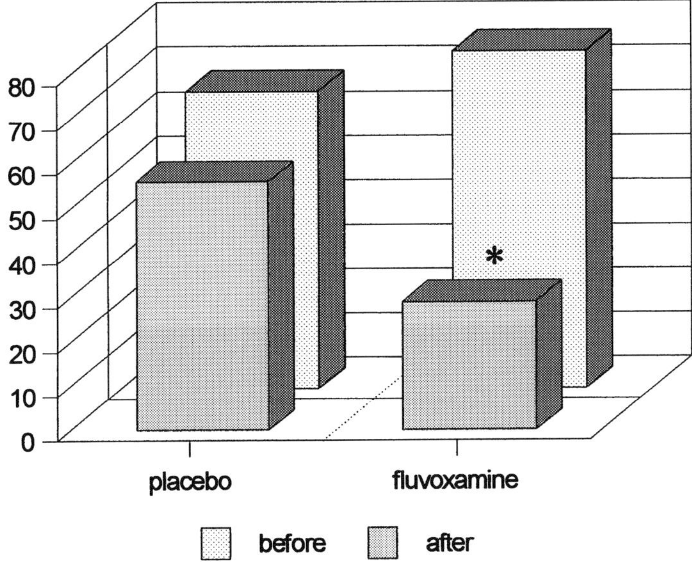

Figure 1. Percentage of panic patients experiencing panic attacks with CCK-4 injection, before and after treatment with placebo or fluvoxamine (reproduced from ref. [16] with kind permission). * Statistically significant (p < 0.01)

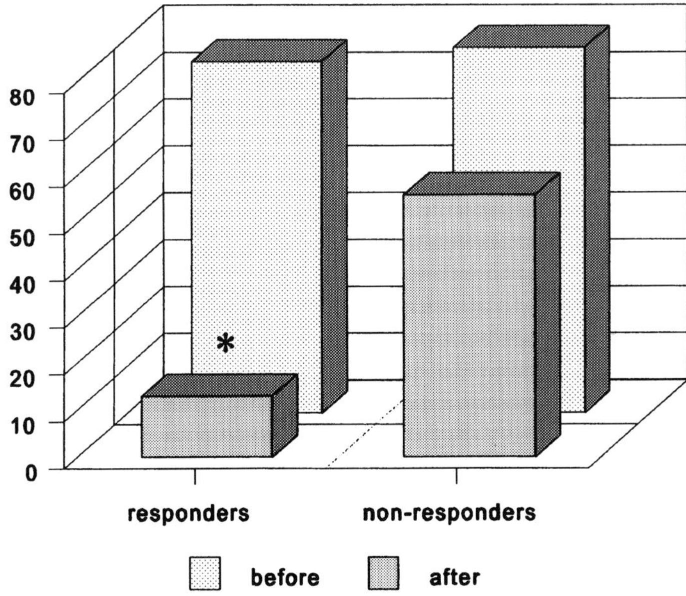

Figure 2. Percentage of panic patients experiencing panic attacks, elicited by CCK-4, before and after treatment with fluvoxamine or placebo. Responders *versus* non-responders (reproduced from ref. [16] with kind permission). * Statistically significant (p < 0.05)

class, known to be effective in panic disorder, decreased the vulnerability of patients suffering with this condition to the panicogenic effect of CCK-4. This effect is not specific to CCK-4 though. Antidepressants also block the effect of other panicogens, e.g. sodium lactate and flumazenil. Following some animal studies [16] and the above data, it is suggested that a functional interaction of 5-HT/CCK-B systems may be at play in panic disorder [4]. However, the evidence is not consistent. Acute depletion of serotonin, using the tryptophan depletion paradigm, failed to alter the panicogenic and cardiovascular effect of CCK-4 in healthy volunteers, although it enhanced the neuroendocrine response of increased ACTH, cortisol and prolactin [17]. Further, there is preliminary evidence showing that the panicogenic effect of cholecystokinin may be mediated through the β adrenergic system. Pre-treatment of normal volunteers with propranolol attenuated the effect of CCK-4, more so than placebo [18]. Since propranolol does not have a central anxiolytic action, this result argues for a peripheral effect of CCK-4.

In an exploratory double-blind study, pre-treatment with L-365,260, a benzodiazepine derivative CCK-B antagonist with very low affinity for CCK-A receptors, prevented the CCK-4 induced panic attacks in patients with panic disorder, in a dose-related fashion [19]. In healthy volunteers, the same drug blocked the panic attacks induced by pentagastrin [20], while CI-988, a peptoid CCK-B antagonist, blocked the panic effect of CCK-4 in a similar population [21], but not in panic disorder patients challenged with CCK-4 [22]. On the contrary, L-365,260 did not affect significantly the panic attacks induced by sodium lactate in panic patients [23], thus indicating a more specific effect in the CCK system. The above show that the CCK-B receptor is unlikely to be the final common receptor mediating panic responses. Nevertheless, the same evidence make it reasonable to expect that CCK antagonists may have a role to play in the treatment of anxiety.

A number of non-peptide CCK-B antagonists, aiming at good blood-brain barrier penetration, oral bioavailability and long duration of action, are under development [24, 4]. However, the clinical trials of CCK-B antagonists have been disappointing so far. A 4-week multi centre, double-blind, placebo-controlled, parallel group study of CI-988 in generalised anxiety disorder (GAD), using a dose of 300 mg daily, was negative. The drug was generally well tolerated. Not surprisingly, the main side-effects were gastrointestinal symptoms. A significant treatment-by-centre interaction and a highly variable placebo response made the interpretation of the results of this study difficult. The authors commented that testing with higher doses of CI-988 may be warranted [25]. Another 6-week multi-centre, placebo-controlled, double-blind study of L-365,260, at a dose of 120 mg daily, in patients with panic disorder with or without agoraphobia, was also negative. This result could not be explained by a high placebo response. The dose, again, may have been suboptimal. There were considerable problems with the preparation of the drug in this study. Its bioavailability and the ability to cross the blood-brain barrier are unknown, thus compromising the results [26].

It is evident from the foregoing discussion that the question about the anxiolytic potential of CCK-B antagonists cannot be answered convincingly yet. Currently, it looks unlikely that drugs acting on CCK receptors alone are effective in treating anxiety [6]. However, in the animal studies where these compounds are successful, they appear to be equally effective as the benzodiazepines, do not produce sedation or muscle relaxation, or interact with alcohol. Further, they do not seem to produce tolerance or dependence, and prevent rebound anxiety occurring from benzodiazepine withdrawal [2]. Therefore, further trials with new compounds are needed to decide whether they have a future as anxiolytics. A number of such drugs are under investigation (e.g. [27–29]).

Corticotropin-releasing factor (CRF)

CRF is a 41 aminoacid peptide, which is produced by the paraventricular nucleus of the hypothalamus (PVN). It is the first relay hormone of the hypothalamo-pituitary-adrenal (HPA) axis, stimulating the release of the basal and stress induced adrenocorticotropin hormone (ACTH). De Souza and Grigoriadis [30] provide an overview of the anatomy of CRF in rat brain. Although the highest concentrations are found in hypothalamus, the peptide is widely distributed in the central nervous system. CRF containing cells are also seen in neocortex, the central nucleus of the amygdala, stria terminalis and substantia inominata. The CRF neurons of the amygdala project to PVN and the parabrachial nucleus of the brainstem, probably affecting both neuroendocrine and autonomic function, as well as behaviour. In the brainstem, CRF neurons are found, among other structures, in the locus coeruleus and the periaqueductal grey matter.

Two G-protein linked CRF receptors have been recognised, named CRF-1 and CRF-2 (with two variants) respectively. In rats, CRF-1 is mostly present in the cortex, limbic system (amygdala, nucleus accumbens, hippocampus), brainstem (locus coeruleus, nucleus tractatus solitarius) and the cerebellum, while CRF-2 appears mainly in subcortical structures, especially the hypothalamus [31]. Following this distribution, the involvement of CRF in cognitive processes, emotion and stress, and autonomic function was postulated [30].

Animal data show that centrally administered CRF is anxiogenic. This effect does not seem to be the result of activation of the pituitary-adrenal axis, since it is not blocked by hypophysectomy. It is probably mediated by CRF receptors above the pituitary level, such as the locus coeruleus [6]. A link with γ-aminobutyric acid (GABA)/benzodiazepine receptor complex has also been hypothesised [32]. In humans, flumazenil, a benzodiazepine receptor antagonist, has been shown to attenuate the ACTH response to CRF, thus indicating a link between the two systems [33]. The results of peptide and nonpeptide CRF antagonists in animal models of anxiety are inconsistent. Some antagonists, while they appear to exert an anxiolytic effect in some models, can produce anxiogenic-like effects in other conditions [6]. It has been suggested that this may depend on the baseline stress level of the animals. A number of studies have indicated that this is a plausible explanation. For example, in non-stressed animals with low endogenous CRF, α-helical CRF-9-41, a CRF fragment which is a CRF receptor antagonist, is anxiogenic. The same compound, used in stressed animals, where endogenous CRF is increased, may produce anxiolytic effects [34].

The evidence that CRF may be involved in the regulation of human anxiety is indirect but considerable. Levels of CRF in the cerebrospinal fluid (CSF) are reportedly high in obsessive-compulsive disorder (OCD) [35] and post-traumatic stress disorder (PTSD) [36], but not in panic disorder [37] or generalised anxiety [38]. Fossey et al. [39] confirmed the higher levels in OCD, but only for male patients, compared with panic, GAD and normal controls. Although the number of subjects in this study was small, it seemed that CRF regulation was affected more by age and gender than diagnosis. CRF levels in recent suicide attempters with mood disorder were significantly lower than controls, irrespective of diagnostic subtype. This could be due either to the depressive illness or to the stress related to the attempt, possibly mediated *via* the negative feedback from increased cortisol levels [40]. Evidence supporting the latter view comes from a study where challenge with intravenous CRF, in patients with a diagnosis of mixed depression and anxiety, showed significantly attenuated ACTH response, compared to patients with depression alone or controls [41]. The two patient groups in this study did not differ in severity of illness. The same challenge in panic [42] and OCD patients [43], revealed a blunted ACTH response compared to controls. This is thought to reflect a process occurring above the pituitary level (see earlier), with stress resulting in endogenous hyper secretion of CRF, which in turn can lead to secondary receptor down regulation in the pituitary and decreased ACTH [44]. These changes in the CRF regulation may be the result of adverse experiences early in life, complementing the genetic predisposition for anxiety disorders [45], or even acting independently to produce a vulnerability for these disorders.

The foregoing results of CRF challenge are not consistent though. A study comparing abused and non-abused depressed children confirmed HPA dysregulation, but ACTH was increased following the administration of CRF, in those children that experienced ongoing chronic adversity. A non-significant trend indicating that children with co-morbid PTSD were more likely to have HPA axis dysregulation than depressed children without PTSD was observed [46]. The authors put forward a number of putative explanations for their findings. Exposure to chronic stress may change the complex feedback mechanisms of the HPA axis in a way that a novel stressor leads to potentiation of CRF effects on pituitary and augmented ACTH response. This may occur at the level of glucocorticoid receptors in hippocampus. Alternatively, it may reflect adaptive changes of monoamine function or arginine vasopressin release from the hypothalamus, with a similar effect on CRF.

A number of CRF receptor antagonists are in various stages of development and testing at present (e.g. [34, 47, 48]). Whether their promised therapeutic potential in human anxiety will be confirmed or not, we should have some hints in the near future.

Neuropeptide Y (NPY)

Neuropeptide Y is a 36 aminoacid peptide, first isolated from mammalian brain tissue in the early 1980s [49]. It belongs to the pancreatic polypeptide family that includes also pancreatic polypeptide (PP) itself and peptide YY (PYY). These are structurally related but functionally diverse peptides. PYY and PP are generally associated with peripheral effects, while NPY is active in the CNS as well [50]. Generally, NPY is co-localised with noradrenaline (NA) [51], while in the central nervous system it also commonly co-exists with GABA and somatostatin [52]. NPY is one of the most powerful stimulants of ingestive behaviour [53]. Other physiological effects of NPY range from regulation of blood pressure, circadian rhythms, and endocrine function, to enhancement of memory retention and anxiolysis [50, 54]. At least some of the above actions, could be accounted for by inhibition of serotonin neurons in the dorsal raphe nuclei, reduction of firing of the locus coeruleus (through potentiation of $\alpha 2$ autoinhibition), as well as potentiation of N-methyl-D-aspartate (NMDA) receptors in hippocampus. In peripheral sympathetic nerves, NPY can inhibit the release of noradrenaline through its presynaptic action, while it potentiates the effect of the same transmitter postsynaptically. These opposing actions are presumably mediated by different NPY receptors (see later) [53, 52]. In the central nervous system NPY is widespread. One *post mortem* human study found the highest concentrations of NPY in the basal ganglia, nucleus accumbens and amygdala, while moderate amounts were seen in the hypothalamus, hippocampus, septal nuclei, cortex and periaqueductal grey matter [55]. As is also the case with other neuropeptides, the distribution of NPY and its binding sites in the brain (see later) are not always co-localised [49].

A number of NPY receptors have been recognised in recent years. They are activated by all three pancreatic polypeptides to a varying degree. The ones that have been cloned so far, Y-1, Y-2, y-6 and Y-5, are linked with G proteins. The first two are found in high densities in the brain. Y-1 and Y-2 also increase intracellular Ca concentrations, while Y-2 can stimulate K channels as well. Y-3, and some other possible variants, are not fully characterised yet. Y-1 receptors are generally thought to be post-synaptic. In the periphery, they are found in blood vessels where they mediate vasoconstriction. In the CNS, they are mainly seen in the cortex, thalamus and amygdala. The latter structure (especially the central nucleus) is linked with NPY's putative anxiolytic effect [56, 50]. Y-2 is thought to be both a postsynaptic and presynaptic receptor, the latter decreasing neurotransmitter release. In the brain, it is mainly found in hippocampus, where it is thought to reduce glutamate release, presumably through a Ca mediation [52]. Y-5, localised in the paraventricular nucleus of the hypothalamus, has been proposed as the "appetite" receptor. Y-4 and y-6 are mainly expressed in the periphery. Y-3 is believed to be present in the brainstem. The study of this class of receptors is still problematic. There is substantial confusion regarding their pharmacological properties and, possibly, their number has been exaggerated [50].

Animal data support the idea that NPY has an anxiolytic effect, while higher levels produce sedation, the latter effect appearing to be unrelated to stimulation of food intake [53]. The antianxiety effect of NPY seems to be mediated by activation of Y-1 receptors, although Y-2 receptors have also been implicated. It is not yet entirely clear whether NPY related anxiolysis is produced through modulation of the function of GABA or NMDA receptor complexes, or noradrenaline neurotransmission. In rats and humans, increased sympathetic activity tends to result in increased plasma levels of NPY [49]. In animal studies, the anxiolytic-like effect of NPY was reversed by the $\alpha2$ adrenergic antagonist idazoxan, but not by the $\alpha1$ antagonist prazosin, or the benzodiazepine receptor antagonist flumazenil [57]. Further, pretreatment with idazoxan also reduced the anxiolytic effect of NPY [58]. These findings suggest that the role NPY is playing in anxiety is related to the regulation of noradrenergic rather than GABAergic transmission, a hypothesis consistent with the co-localisation of NPY and NA in the nervous system [49]. It has also been proposed that NPY may act as an endogenous buffer against the stress-induced CRF release in the amygdala, thus exerting its anxiolytic effect through this mechanism [59].

In humans, low levels of CSF neuropeptide Y were associated with loss of appetite and anorexia nervosa [60, 61]. There is also emerging clinical evidence that NPY may be involved in the regulation of stress and anxiety. CSF concentrations of NPY in depressed patients, were negatively correlated with their anxiety scores. The level of NPY tended to decrease as anxiety scores increased [62]. Further indirect evidence was produced by a *post mortem* study of suicide victims, which showed reduced concentrations of NPY, especially in frontal regions, compared to subjects that died naturally or accidentally [63]. Recent suicide attempters with mood disorder, especially those with repeated attempts, had lower plasma NPY levels compared with controls. Whether this is related to the mood disorder or the underlying stress associated with the attempt remains unclear. In the same study, dexamethasone suppressed NPY levels in controls, but not in patients [40]. In an attempt to look at the relationship of NPY with noradrenaline (NA) and anxiety more closely, Rasmusson et al. [51] studied healthy volunteers, in a double-blind placebo-controlled fashion, using yohimbine (0.4 mg/kg), an $\alpha2$ antagonist known to induce anxiety and increase plasma NA. Plasma NPY and 3-methyl-4-hydroxyphenylglycol (MHPG) (the main NA metabolite) levels were significantly increased after yohimbine treatment. There was also a positive correlation between the percent change of plasma NPY and MHPG in response to yohimbine. This is consistent with the view that NPY and NA are extensively co-localised in the central nervous system. These results were at odds though with a previous study [64], in which plasma NA increased substantially but NPY did not change after yohimbine challenge. The most likely explanation is that the dose of yohimbine used in this study was too low, i.e. 0.25 mg/kg, since yohimbine-stimulated NPY release is thought to be dose-dependent [51]. However, it should be borne in mind that plasma NPY levels are affected by a variety of factors, such as the subject being in upright or prone position during venepuncture, differential metabolism between subjects depending on their psychopathology, and recent levels of physical activity [40]. These variations make the interpretation of the above results problematic.

Following the above clinical evidence and the available animal data, it has been hypothesised that NPY regulates human anxiety *via* its effect on nora-drenergic transmission [51]. However, direct studies of NPY levels in anxiety disorders have yielded inconsistent results. Boulenger et al. [65] found higher plasma NPY levels in panic patients compared with healthy volunteers, a find-ing not replicated by Stein et al. [66]. In this latter study, baseline plasma lev-els of NPY did not differ between patients with panic disorder, social phobia, and healthy volunteers. The levels of NPY did not correlate with that of NA either, although, in panic patients only, it was observed that baseline NPY lev-els correlated negatively with anxiety scores. Following exposure to the acute stress of the cold pressor test (immersion of one hand in ice water for 3 min) NA levels increased and NPY levels fell, but, again, there was no difference between the various groups. Finally, the NPY and NA levels, after exposure to the stressful situation, did not correlate with the intensity of anxiety symptoms. The reasons for these discrepant results are not known. Further evaluation of the role of NPY in human anxiety is warranted, perhaps by using different provocative stimuli, such as prolonged physical exercise or insulin-induced hypoglycaemia, which are known to elicit NPY release [66].

The study of NPY will be further advanced once non-peptide agonists and receptor selective antagonists of NPY receptors become available [49]. Efforts to develop NPY receptor ligands have not been fruitful yet [53], but they con-tinue unabated [67, 68]. Their future usefulness as anxiolytics is therefore still only a theoretical possibility. Because of the lack of specific ligands, Wahlestedt and his colleagues [56] employed a novel approach, the antisense technique, in order to study the role of endogenous NPY in anxiety, in the liv-ing rat brain. They constructed an antisense oligodeoxynucleotide correspon-ding to the rat Y-1 receptor. This oligodeoxynucleotide was then repeatedly injected into the lateral cerebral ventricles of the animals. Subsequently, the antisense treated animals were subjected to a stress model, and they showed marked behavioral signs of anxiety, compared with the control animals. *Post mortem* of the antisense treated rat brains showed that this technique achieved a 60% reduction of cortical Y-1 receptors, without affecting the number of Y-2 receptors. However interesting and important in elucidating the neurobiology of anxiety, the antisense technique is not a viable route for treatment.

Substance P

Substance P was discovered in 1931 by von Euler and Gaddum. It is the most abundant of the neurokinin (tachykinin) group of peptides, that also includes neurokinin A and neuromedin K [69]. It is a major transmitter of small, unmyelinated, primary afferent nerves of the substantia gelatinosa of the spinal cord and the spinal tract of the trigeminal nerve, where it exerts a primary role in pain transmission. Stimulation of substance P fibres produces burning pain. In the central nervous system, substance P neurons are present in medullary tegmental nuclei, the central nucleus of amygdala and, notably, in the spiny neurons of the striatum that project to the medial segment of the globus pallidus and the substantia nigra pars reticulata. Fewer substance P neurons are present in the dentate gyrus of hippocampus. Some neurons are also present in layers 5 and 6 of the cortex, where they seem to project to the upper layers [70].

The three recognised neurokinin receptors are coupled by G proteins and they are named NK-1, NK-2 and NK-3 respectively. Of these NK-1 is the substance P preferring receptor. It is widely distributed both in the periphery and the central nervous system, mainly the dorsal horn of the spinal cord, the olfactory bulb and the striatum [70], as well as areas traditionally implicated in fear and anxiety, i.e. the hypothalamus, the amygdala, the hippocampus and the periaqueductal grey matter [71]. Similar to other neuropeptides, e.g. the opiates and NPY, there is considerable divergence between the location of these peptides and their receptors [70].

NK-1/substance P antagonists have been investigated for many years as potential agents in pain relief. Early attempts were hampered by the poor bioavailability of antagonists resembling substance P itself. The development of smaller molecule antagonists in recent years gave new impetus in this area of research. It has been suggested that, apart from pain, the NK-1 antagonists may have a role to play in a number of conditions such as inflammation, asthma, emesis, migraine, depression and anxiety [69]. Several studies have investigated substance P and NK-1 antagonists in animal models of anxiety. There is enough evidence to suggest a role for substance P in the modulation of anxiety, although its effects appear to be dependent on dose and specific brain region. Consequently, the results with specific NK-1 antagonists are variable and contradictory [6]. There is also some evidence from animal studies supporting the notion that NK-2 antagonists may have an anxiolytic profile [2].

The limited human data of Substance P receptor ligands are encouraging so far. MK-869, an NK-1 antagonist, has recently been tested in the treatment of moderate to severe depression. In clinical trials in four sites, the experimental drug was used at a single dose of 300 mg daily and its effect was comparable to a moderate clinical dose of paroxetine, i.e. 20 mg daily, and significantly better than placebo. The drug was safe and well tolerated [72]. This effect appears to be independent of any augmentation of serotonin or noradrenaline function, but the fact that the efficacy of MK-869 was expressed 2–3 weeks following the onset of treatment suggests the possibility of a final common pathway for the action of antidepressants [69]. From week 4 onwards the two active drugs, MK-869 and paroxetine, also reduced anxiety, measured with the Hamilton anxiety scale, significantly more so than placebo (Fig. 3). Given the effectiveness of serotonin reuptake inhibitors, such as paroxetine used in this trial, in a range of anxiety conditions, the above results offer a realistic chance that substance P antagonists like MK-869 will prove effective in anxiety disorders [73]. A number of such antagonists are under development (e.g. [29, 74]).

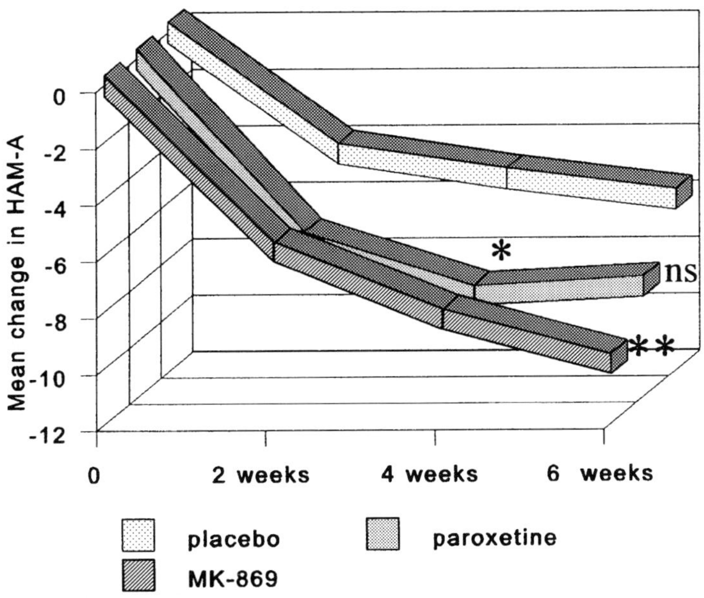

Figure 3. Change in Hamilton Anxiety Scale (HAM-A) scores in depressed patients treated with the substance P antagonist MK-869, paroxetine and placebo (from ref. [72]). $^*p \leq 0.05$, $^{**}p \leq 0.002$, ns: not significant. (Reprinted with permission from Kramer et al. (1998) *Science* 281: 1640–1645 [72]. Copyright 2000 American Association for the Advancement of Science.)

Endorphins

The endorphins (enkephalins and dynorphins) are endogenous compounds that have activity at the opiate receptors. They are synthetised by cleavage of larger peptide precursors. Both enkephalin and dynorphin containing neurons appear as local interneurons in the primary sensory areas of the dorsal horn of the spinal cord and the spinal tract of the trigeminal nucleus, where they serve to suppress pain sensation. They are also widely distributed in the brain, with particularly high concentrations in the striatum, the central grey and periaqueductal gray matter, the central nucleus of the amygdala and other areas [70].

Three specific sites for opiate binding have been characterised, the γ, δ and κ receptors. The first is the substrate for opiate analgesics. δ receptors are more specific for enkephalins and k receptors for dynorphins. The distribution of these ligand binding sites in the brain is very different from the distribution of the peptide containing nerve terminals. The same paradox is true of many other peptide neurotransmitters and neuromodulators. This conundrum is still unresolved. Perhaps, the peptides diffuse over long distances to stimulate the receptors. On the other hand, presence of the peptide may down regulate its receptor population. Finally, the peptide transmitters may be paradoxically present in areas where they have no functional role [70].

The narcotic opioids are the most efficacious of all anxiolytics. Because of their high dependence and abuse potential they are not used in this context. The high prevalence of neurotic illness in addicts [75] suggests that at least some of them may be using opioids for this indication. It is theoretically possible that a weak partial agonist of μ receptors would retain the anxiolytic properties of the full agonists but not produce the euphoria to lead to abuse. An alternative strategy would be to reduce the dysphoric tone produced by the endogenous κ agonists, dynorphins [76].

Somatostatin (SS)

Somatostatin appears as a family of peptides, the commonest biologically active form being a tetradecapeptide. In the gut it inhibits insulin, while in the brain it exerts a similar effect on the growth hormone (GH) release. In conjunction with CCK (see earlier) its discovery proved pivotal in the recognition that gut peptides are also present in the brain. Abnormal SS activity has been postulated in a variety of psychiatric disorders [77]. Significantly elevated CSF levels of SS were reported in obsessive-compulsive patients compared to controls [78], but not in panic disorder [79]. Given that serotonergic antidepressants are the treatment of choice in OCD and are also extensively used in panic, the finding in rats that these agents decrease SS [80] is potentially very interesting. A small series of panic patients treated with a long-acting somatostatin analogue experienced significant relief from their symptoms [81]. However, there is some evidence that SS levels in adulthood may be the result of adverse early rearing experiences [82], thus pointing towards a trait rather than a state phenomenon. Therefore, the relationship between somatostatin and anxiety states needs to be further disentangled before rational design of drugs can proceed.

Angiotensin

The angiotensin-converting enzyme (ACE) inhibitors, such as captopril, are used in medicine to treat hypertension. They inhibit the conversion of angiotensin I (AI) to the octapeptide angiotensin II (AII). Both in animal and some human studies they show an anxiolytic profile, in some cases comparable with that of the benzodiazepines [2]. The mechanism by which this effect is mediated remains unclear. There is some animal evidence that AII-1 and AII-2 receptors may be involved in this action and the regulation of anxiety in general. The picture is still confusing though. Mice lacking AII receptors exhibited anxiety-like behaviour [83], but angiotensin did not seem to influence anxiety behaviour in mice under normal conditions [84]. In one study, an AII antagonist showed anxiolytic effects in rats [85], but, in another study, both AI and AII antagonists gave negative results [86]. The involvement of noradrenergic [83] and serotonergic [87] systems in the effect of angiotensin on anxiety has been postulated. Clearly, a lot more basic research is needed in this area for a consistent picture to emerge.

Galanin

Galanin is a 29 aminoacid peptide, which is functionally related to neuropeptide Y. It is widely expressed in the central nervous system, and a role has been suggested for this peptide in memory function, food intake and endocrine control. Its receptors are linked to G proteins. The involvement of galanin in the regulation of anxiety was postulated after it was found in areas like the amygdala, and locus coeruleus. Despite its presence in this principal nucleus of noradrenaline containing neurons, it is not yet known to what extent the two transmitters co-exist. Galanin appears to interact with serotonergic neurons as well. In a study in rats, centrally administered galanin produced an anxiolytic effect, albeit lower than that of benzodiazepines or of neuropeptide Y [88]. Galanin has not been widely studied yet. Further, the little information that is available to date is based on animal studies. A role for ligands of the receptors of this peptide in anxiety treatment cannot be excluded though.

Thyrotropin releasing hormone (TRH)

This tripeptide is produced in the hypothalamus and regulates the release of thyroid stimulating hormone (TSH) from the anterior pituitary. It may also stimulate prolactin release, while an effect on growth hormone (GH) and ACTH is absent in normal subjects but present in various pathological conditions. TRH containing cells are also present in many CNS areas, amongst others the hippocampus, amygdala, nucleus accumbens, periaqueductal grey matter, paraventricular nucleus, substantia nigra and raphe nuclei. The central effects of this peptide are not mediated by its endocrine effects. TRH co-exists in the brain with other transmitters and modulators, such as serotonin, dopamine, histamine, neuropeptide Y, substance P, and the enkephalins. TRH receptors belong to the G protein group [89].

In animal studies of anxiety, TRH appears to augment the anxiolytic-like effect of benzodiazepines and alcohol, and in higher doses it shows an anxiolytic effect itself [89]. Conversely, benzodiazepines have been shown to inhibit TSH and prolactin release in animals, following exposure to stress. However, 1 week pre-treatment with diazepam did not alter TRH-induced TSH response in a small sample of patients with GAD or adjustment disorder. By contrast TRH-induced prolactin release was decreased [90]. In other animal studies, stress elicits TRH release, which is blocked by ipsapirone, a 5-HT-1a agonist, thus indicating an interaction with the serotonin systems in the brain [91].

In humans, TRH has been extensively studied in depression, where a blunted response of TSH following TRH stimulation has been reported in 25–30% of patients [89]. Although similar findings have been reported for panic, other studies failed to detect an effect of TRH on TSH levels in this condition [92]. Challenge with TRH in panic disorder did not produce a different GH response compared to healthy controls either [93]. In fact, although the subjects experienced palpitations, nausea and paraesthesias, only 5% had a panic attack with 0.5 mg of TRH. This argues against the cognitive theory of panic disorder, which postulates that panic attacks are generated following misinterpretation of peripheral somatic symptoms of autonomic origin. Similarly, TRH challenge in social phobia gave negative results [94]. This may be explained by the use of a dose which is not comparable to other panicogenics, such as pentagastrin [95]. However, PTSD sufferers did show blunted TSH response to TRH. Treatment of this group with desipramine improved the depression levels substantially, but failed to affect PTSD, other anxiety symptoms, or the TSH response to TRH [96]. In a study of 45 patients with panic, GAD and OCD, Fossey et al. [97] found no difference in the CSF concentration of TRH of the patient group compared to nonpsychiatric controls.

There are major difficulties in the study of the therapeutic use of TRH in human anxiety. The half-life of the peptide is very short (<5 min) and it causes significant (albeit transient) increase in blood pressure. The first problem can be solved with the development of longer lasting stable analogues of TRH, and some have already been tested, although oral bioavailability remains an issue. These analogues tend to share the cardiovascular effects of the original hormone [98]. Single dose of 0.5 mg synthetic TRH (protirelin) showed a rapid and robust antidepressant effect, with significant reduction of suicidality. However, this effect was short lived and, in order to overcome the poor blood-brain barrier permeability, the drug was given *via* a lumbar intrathecal injection. This renders its therapeutic use impractical [99]. Single dose 0.2 mg intravenous administration of protirelin in depressed women also elevated mood rapidly, but the effect was more evident in patients without associated panic attacks than in patients with panic [100]. The peripheral anxiety-like symptoms that healthy volunteers experienced, as mentioned earlier, suggest that TRH may be in fact anxiogenic. In some of the depression studies though, an improvement in anxiety was observed with the TRH challenge [89]. Hence, to draw any conclusions about the involvement of TRH in the regulation of human anxiety and its potential therapeutic use would be premature.

Arginine vasopressin (AVP) and oxytocin (OT)

Vasopressin and oxytocin are two related nonapeptides found exclusively in mammals. After they are produced in the hypothalamus, mainly in the supraoptic and paraventricular nuclei, they are released in the circulation from the neurohypophysis. In the periphery, AVP enables the kidneys to retain water in conditions of dehydration, while in much higher levels it produces vaso-constriction. OT facilitates parturition and release of milk from the mammary glands through muscle contraction. AVP and OT neurons also project from hypothalamus to the rest of the central nervous system. The presence of extra-hypothalamic neurons containing these peptides has also been shown. A number of central functions have been studied in relation to these neuropeptides, including memory and ingestive behaviour [101].

AVP is released within the rat paraventricular nucleus in response to emotional stress and it has been hypothesised that this release provides a negative feedback on the HPA axis [102]. Centrally administered AVP has an anxiogenic effect in rats, an effect blocked by the dopamine D2 antagonist pimozide [103]. Although this finding is not consistent, a vasopressin V1 receptor antagonist seems to have an anxiolytic-like effect [104], and antisense treatment of the same receptor also reduced anxiety related behaviour. The area involved in this action of vasopressin is thought to be the septum [105].

Limited data are available from humans. In OCD, baseline vasopressin CSF levels have been reported either elevated [106] or not different compared with controls [107]. On the other hand, treatment of OCD with clomipramine reduced AVP levels in the cerebrospinal fluid [35]. The interpretation of these results, especially in conjunction with the oxytocin results (see later), is not very clear.

Animal studies show that oxytocin has an anxiolytic effect. It appears to affect both behavioural and endocrine responses to stress [108]. By reducing anxiety, OT is thought to increase socialising [109]. The anxiolytic effect of OT seems to be mediated *via* 5-HT-1a receptor mechanisms [110]. 5-HT-1a is both a pre- and postsynaptic receptor. Presynaptic 5-HT-1a is an autoreceptor, which reduces the firing of the 5-HT neuron, therefore inhibiting the release of serotonin. It has been implicated in the regulation of anxiety, and drugs acting on this receptor have an anxiolytic profile, e.g. buspirone. It is also suggested that the anxiolytic effects of the SSRIs are mediated *via* the same receptor, as a result of its desensitisation, following chronic treatment. Citalopram, an SSRI, increases oxytocin levels in rats and there appears to be little or no tolerance to this effect [111]. In view of the therapeutic use of serotonergic drugs in anxiety disorders, the above findings, linking OT with the serotonin system, are potentially very interesting. The human data with this peptide are limited to OCD so far. In one study CSF oxytocin levels were markedly higher in patients compared with controls and they correlated significantly with symptom severity [107]. However, Altemus et al. [112] failed to replicate this result. Methodological differences between the studies, and a smaller sample size in the negative one, may have accounted for this discrepancy. Swedo et al. [113] found no correlation between CSF oxytocin levels and symptom severity in children and adolescent OCD patients. However, long-term treatment of OCD with clomipramine further increased CSF oxytocin levels [35]. This may reflect reduced postsynaptic OT receptor sensitivity and decreased negative feedback to the OT system in the brain. Therefore the initial elevation during the illness period may be compensatory in nature, while higher levels of this neuropeptide may also play a role in recovery. Indeed, the therapeutic action of clomipramine may be mediated through oxytocin. On the other hand, these differences in OT levels in illness and after recovery may indicate a trait and state phenomenon. Clearly, more studies in anxiety disorders other than OCD are needed in this area, especially in social phobia. The full characterisation of the oxytocin receptors in the brain and the development of analogues for these receptors is a potentially very interesting avenue for future anxiolytic treatments.

Summary and conclusion

The study of neuropeptides in anxiety has been a very active area of research in recent years. Despite the considerable advances in our knowledge, and the early excitement and promise, little has been achieved so far in this area by means of producing new effective treatments (Tab. 1). While some of the problems, such as poor bioavailability of compounds, may be solved in the near future, more questions have been generated regarding the relative role of various transmitters and modulators in regulating human anxiety. The way forward probably stems from better understanding of the relationship between neuropeptides and classical neurotransmitters in general and in specific areas of the brain implicated in psychopathology.

Research on this topic has been, so far, conducted mainly in animals. For example, serotonin interacts extensively with neuropeptides. There are reports that CCK, CRF, neuropeptide Y, substance P and galanin may alter 5-HT synthesis. Serotonin, on the other hand, may stimulate the release of CRF in paraventricular nucleus of the hypothalamus and other areas of the brain. Further, serotonin co-exists with other neuropeptides, such as enkephalin, somatostatin and substance P [114]. In the striatum, animal data suggest that, although the principal transmitter of the substance P/dynorphin neurons projecting to substantia nigra, and the enkephalin neurons, projecting to the globus pallidus, is GABA, these neurons are also under regulation by dopamine transmission [1]. By the same token, electrophysiological animal studies indicate that CCK not

Table 1. Evidence for the involvement of various neuropeptides and their receptor ligands in the regulation of anxiety

	Animals	Humans
CCK/pentagastrin	↑ (++)*	↑ (++)
CCK antagonists	↓ (++)	ne
CRF	↑ (++)	↑ (+)
CRF antagonists	↑ ↓ (?)*	nd
NPY/Y-1 agonism	↓ (++)	↓ (?+)
Substance P/NK1 antagonists	↓ (+)	↓ (?+)
Endorphins/μ agonists	↓ (+)	↓ (+)
Somatostatin	↓ (+)	↓ (+)
Angiotensin	?	↓ (?+)
Angiotensin AII antagonists	↓ (?+)	nd
Galanin	↓ (+)	nd
TRH & analogues	↑ ↓ (?)	↑ ↓ (?)
Vasopressin	↑ (?+)	?
AVP antagonists	↓ (+)	nd
Oytocin	↓ (+)	↓ (?+)

↑: increase in anxiety
↓: decrease in anxiety
++: strong evidence
+: positive evidence
?+: positive evidence, but not consistent
?: contradictory evidence
ne: negative evidence
nd: not done
*: dependent upon baseline levels of anxiety

only promotes the utilisation and/or metabolism of serotonin but it also interacts extensively with GABA [4]. The relative interaction between various neuropeptide systems may be also very important. For instance, the balance between CRF and NPY appears to affect the regulation of sleep and arousal in rats. It has been suggested that disturbance of this ratio may underlie the dysregulation of these functions in depression and anxiety [54]. The interplay with hormones should also be taken into account. In the study described earlier, where CRF and NPY plasma levels were lower in recent suicide attempters compared to controls, cortisol was found to be elevated in the patient population. The CRF and NPY levels could be reduced as a result of high cortisol levels, induced by prolonged stress [40].

What the above illustrates is the complexity of the regulation of chemical transmission in the central nervous system. Perhaps, the most important contribution of the neuropeptide study, so far, has been to dispel the simplistic idea that one single transmitter may be responsible for as wide a phenomenon as anxiety. The idea that each transmitter can modify the response of neurons to its co-transmitters is gaining popularity [114], but it opens a seemingly infinite repertoire of combinations, which may look bewildering. The clarification of these complex inter-relationships though may shed some light to the pathophysiology of anxiety and lead to better designed treatments.

References

1 Hökfelt TGM, Castel M-N, Morino P, Zhang X, Dagerlind A (1995) General overview of neuropeptides. *In*: FE Bloom, DJ Kupfer (eds): *Psychopharmacology. The fourth generation of progress*. Raven Press, New York, 483–492

2 Jackson HC, Nutt DJ (1995) Anxiety and panic disorders. *In*: L Pullan, J Patel (eds): *Neurotherapeutics: emerging strategies. Basic and clinical perspectives*. Humana Press, New Jersey, 85–131

3 Pearse AGE (1966) 5-hydroxy-tryptophan uptake by dog thyroid C cells and its possible significance in polypeptide hormone production. *Nature* 211: 598–600

4 van Megen HJGM, Westenberg HGM, den Boer JA, Kahn RS (1996) Cholecystokinin in anxiety. *Eur Neuropsychopharmacol* 6: 263–280

5 Vanderhaegen JJ, Signeau JC, Gepts W (1975) New peptide in the vertebrate CNS reacting with antigastrin antibodies. *Nature* 257: 604–605

6 Griebel G (1999) Is there a future for neuropeptide receptor ligands in the treatment of anxiety disorders? *Pharmacol Ther* 82: 1–61

7 Shlik J, Zhou Y, Koszycki D, Vaccarino FJ, Bradwejn J (1999) Effects of CCK-4 infusion on the acoustic eye-blink startle and psychophysiological measures in healthy volunteers. *J Psychopharmacol* 13: 385–390

8 de Montigny C (1989) Cholecystokinin tetrapeptide induces panic-like attacks in healthy volunteers. *Arch Gen Psychiat* 46: 511–517

9 De Leeuw A, den Boer JA, Slaap BR, Westenberg HGMJA (1996) Pentagastrin has panic-inducing properties in obsessive compulsive disorder. *Psychopharmacology* 126: 339–344

10 Brawman-Mintzer O, Lydiard RB, Bradwejn J, Villareal G, Knapp R, Emmanuel N, Ware MR, He Q, Ballenger JC (1997) Effects of the cholecystokinin agonist pentagastrin in patients with generalised anxiety disorder. *Amer J Psychiat* 154: 700–702

11 van Vliet IM, Westenberg HGM, Slaap BR, den Boer JA, Ho-Pian KL (1997) Anxiogenic effects of pentagastrin in patients with social phobia and healthy controls. *Biol Psychiat* 42: 76–78

12 Javanmard M, Shlik J, Kennedy SH, Vaccarino FJ, Houle S, Bradwejn J (1999) Neuroanatomic correlates of CCK-4 induced panic attacks in healthy humans: a comparison of two time points. *Biol Psychiat* 45: 872–882

13 Malizia AL, Nutt DJ (1999) Brain mechanisms and circuits in panic disorder. *In*: DJ Nutt, JC Ballenger, JP Lepine (eds): *Panic disorder. Clinical diagnosis, management and mechanisms*. Martin Dunitz, London, 55–77

14 Malizia AL (1999) What do brain imaging studies tell us about anxiety disorders? *J Psychopharmacol* 13: 372–378

15 Bradwejn J, Koszycki D (1994) Imipramine antagonism of the panicogenic effects of cholecystokinin tetrapeptide in panic disorder patients. *Amer J Psychiat* 151: 261–263

16 van Megen HJGM, Westenberg HGM, den Boer JA, Slaap B, Scheepmarkers A (1997) Effect of the selective serotonin reuptake inhibitor fluvoxamine on CCK-4 induced panic attacks. *Psychopharmacology* 129: 357–364

17 Koszycki D, Zacharko RM, Le Melledo J-M, Young SN, Bradwejn J (1996) Effect of acute tryptophan depletion on behavioural, cardiovascular, and hormonal sensitivity to cholecystokinin-tetrapeptide challenge in healthy volunteers. *Biol Psychiat* 40: 648–655

18 Le Melledo J-M, Bradwejn J, Koszycki D, Bichet DG, Bellavance F (1998) The role of the β-noradrenergic system in cholecystokinin-tetrapeptide-induced panic symptoms. *Biol Psychiat* 44: 364–366

19 Bradwejn J, Koszycki D, Couteaux du Tertre A, van Megen H, den Boer JA, Westenberg H (1994) The panicogenic effects of cholecystokinin tetrapeptide are antagonised by L-365,260, a central

cholecystokinin receptor antagonist in patients with panic disorder. *Arch Gen Psychiat* 51: 486–493

20 Lines C, Challenor J, Traub M (1995) Cholecystokinin and anxiety in normal volunteers: an investigation of the anxiogenic properties of pentagastrin and reversal by cholecystokinin receptor subtype B antagonist L-365,260. *Brit J Pharmacol* 39: 235–242

21 Bradwejn J, Koszycki D, Paradis M, Reece P, Hinton J, Sedman A (1995) Effect of CI-988 on cholecystokinin tetrapeptide-induced panic symptoms in healthy volunteers. *Biol Psychiat* 10: 27–42

22 van Megen HJ, Westenberg HG, den Boer JA, Slaap B, van Es Radhakishua F, Pande AC (1997) The cholecystokinin-B receptor antagonist CI-988 failed to affect CCK-4 induced symptoms in panic disorder patients. *Psychopharmacology* 129: 243–248

23 van Megen HJGM, Westenberg HGM, den Boer JA (1996) Effect of the cholecystokinin-B (CCK-B) receptor antagonist L-365,260 on lactate induced panic attacks in panic disorder patients. *Biol Psychiat* 40: 804–806

24 Mosconi M, Chiamulera C, Recchia G (1993) New anxiolytics in development. *Int J Clin Pharm Res* 6: 331–344

25 Adams JB, Pyke RE, Costa J, Cutler NR, Scweizer E, Wilcox CS, Wisselink PG, Greiner M, Pierre MW, Pande AC (1995) A double-blind, placebo-controlled study of a CCK-B antagonist, CI-988, in patients with generalised anxiety disorder. *J Clin Psychopharmacol* 15: 428–434

26 Kramer MS, Cutler NR, Ballenger JC, Patterson WM, Mendels J, Chenault A, Shrivastava R, Matzura-Wolfe D, Lines C, Reines S (1995) A placebo-controlled trial of L-365,260, a CCK-B antagonist, in panic disorder. *Biol Psychiat* 37: 462–466

27 Trivedi BK, Padia JK, Holmes A, Rose S, Wright DS, Hinton JP, Pritchard MC, Eden JM, Kneen C, Webdale L et al (1998) Second generation «peptoid» CCK-B receptor antagonists: identification and development of N-(adamantyloxycarbonyl)-alpha-methyl-(R)-tryptophan derivative (CI-1015) with an improved pharmacokinetic profile. *J Med Chem* 41: 38–45

28 Semple G, Ryder H, Rooker DP, Batt AR, Kendrick DA, Szelke M, Ohta M, Satoh M, Nishida A, Akuzawa S et al (1997) (3R)-N-(1-(tert-butylcarbonylmethyl)-2,3-dihydro-2-oxo-5-(2-pyridyl)-1H-1,4-benzodiazepin-3-yl)-N=-(3-(methylamino)phenyl)urea (YF476): a potent and orally active gastrin/CCK-B antagonist. *J Med Chem* 40: 331–341

29 Horwell D, Pritchard M, Raphy J, Ratcliffe G (1996) Targeted molecular diversity: design and development of non-peptide antagonists for cholecystokinin and tachykinin receptors. *Immunopharmacology* 33: 68–72

30 De Souza EB, Grigoriadis DE (1995) Corticotropin-Releasing Factor. *In*: FE Bloom, DJ Kupfer (eds): *Psychopharmacology. The fourth generation of progress*. Raven Press, New York, 505–517

31 Chalmers DT, Lovenberg TW, De Souza EB (1995) Localization of novel corticotropin-releasing factor receptor (CRF-2) mRNA expression to specific subcortical nuclei in rat brain: comparison with CRF-1 receptor mRNA expression. *J Neurosci* 15: 6340–6350

32 Kunovac JL, Stahl SM (1995) Future directions in anxiolytic pharmacotherapy. *Psychit Clin N Amer* 18: 895–909

33 Ströhle A, Wiedemann K (1996) Flumazenil attenuates the pituitary response to CRH in healthy males. *Eur Neuropsychopharmacol* 6: 323–325

34 Menzaghi F, Howard RL, Heinrichs SC, Vale W, Rivier J, Koob GF (1994) Characterisation of a novel and potent corticotropin-releasing factor antagonist in rats. *J Pharmacol Exp Ther* 269: 564–572

35 Altemus M, Swedo SE, Leonard HL, Richter D, Rubinow DR, Murphy DL, Gold PW (1994) Changes in cerebrospinal fluid neurochemistry during treatment of obsessive-compulsive disorder with clomipramine. *Arch Gen Psychiat* 51: 794–803

36 Bremner JD, Licinio J, Darnell A, Krystal JH, Owens MJ, Southwick SM, Nemeroff CB, Charney DS (1997) Elevated CSF corticotropin-releasing factor concentrations in posttraumatic stress disorder. *Amer J Psychiat* 154: 624–629

37 Jolkkonen J, Lepola U, Bissette G, Nemeroff C, Riekkinen P (1993) CSF corticotropin-releasing factor is not affected in panic disorder. *Biol Psychiat* 33: 136–138

38 Banki CM, Karmacsi L, Bissette G, Nemeroff CB (1992) Cerebrospinal fluid neuropeptides in mood disorder and dementia. *J Affect Disord* 25: 39–45

39 Fossey MD, Lydiard RB, Ballenger JC, Laraia MT, Bissette G, Nemeroff CB (1996) Cerebrospinal fluid corticotropin-releasing factor concentrations in patients with anxiety disorders and normal comparison subjects. *Biol Psychiat* 39: 703–707

40 Westrin Å, Ekman R, Träskman-Benz L (1999) Alterations of corticotropin releasing hormone (CRH) and neuropeptide Y (NPY) plasma levels in mood disorder patients with recent suicide attempt. *Eur Neuropsychopharmacol* 9: 205–211

41 Meller WH, Kathol RG, Samuelson SD, Gehris TL, Carroll BT, Pitts AF, Clayton PJ (1995) CRH challenge test in anxious depression. *Biol Psychiat* 37: 376–382

42 Roy Byrne PP, Uhde TW, Post RM, Gallucci W, Chrousos GP, Gold PW (1986) The corticotropin-releasing hormone stimulation test in patients with panic disorder. *Amer J Psychiat* 143: 896–899

43 Servant D (1997) Role of corticotropin-releasing factor in anxiety. *Biol Psychiat* 42: 60–65

44 De Souza EB (1995) Corticotropin-releasing factor receptors: physiology, pharmacology, biochemistry and role in central nervous system and immune disorders. *Psychoneuroendocrinology* 20: 789–819

45 Heim C, Owens MJ, Plotsky PM, Nemeroff CB (1997) Persistent changes in corticotropin-releasing factor systems due to early life stress: relationships to the pathophysiology of major depression and post-traumatic stress disorder. *Psychopharmacol Bull* 33: 185–192

46 Kaufman J, Birmaher B, Perel J, Dahl RE, Moreci P, Nelson B, Wells W, Ryan ND (1997) The corticotropin-releasing hormone challenge in depressed abused, depressed nonabused, and normal control children. *Biol Psychiat* 42: 669–679

47 Griebel G, Perrault G, Sanger DJ (1998) Characterization of the behavioural profile of the non-peptide CRF receptor antagonist CP-154,526 in anxiety model in rodents. Comparison with diazepam and buspirone. *Psychopharmacology* 138: 55–66

48 Kask A, Rago L, Harro J (1997) Alpha-helical CRF(9–41) prevents anxiogenic-like effect of NPY Y-1 receptor antagonist BIBP3226 in rats. *Neuroreport* 8: 3645–3647

49 Wettstein JG, Earley B, Junien JL (1995) Central nervous system pharmacology of neuropeptide Y. *Pharmacol Ther* 65: 397–414

50 Blomqvist AG, Herzog H (1997) Y-receptor subtypes – how many more? *Trends Neurosci* 20: 294–298

51 Rasmusson AM, Southwick SM, Hauger RL, Charney DS (1998) Plasma neuropeptide Y (NPY) increases in humans in response to the a2 antagonist yohimbine. *Neuropsychopharmacology* 19: 95–98

52 Munglani R, Hundspith MJ, Hunt SP (1996) The therapeutic potential of neuropeptide Y. *Drugs* 52: 371–389

53 Grundemar L, Håkanson R (1994) Neuropeptide Y effector systems: perspectives for drug development. *Trends Pharmacol Sci* 15: 153–159

54 Ehlers CL, Somes C, Seifritz E, Rivier JE (1997) CRF/NPY interactions: a potential role in sleep dysregulation in depression and anxiety. *Depress Anxiety* 6: 1–9

55 Adrian TE, Allen JM, Bloom SR, Ghatei MA, Rossor MN, Roberts GW, Crow TJ, Tatemoto K, Pollak JM (1983) Neuropeptide Y distribution in human brain. *Nature* 306: 584–586

56 Wahlestedt C, Merlo Pich M, Koob GF, Yee F, Heilig M (1993) Modulation of anxiety and neuropeptide Y/Y-1 receptors by antisense oligodeoxynucleotides. *Science* 259: 528–531

57 Heilig M, Wahlestedt C, Widerlöv E (1988) Neuropeptide Y (NPY) induced suppression of activity in the rat: evidence for NPY receptor heterogeneity and for interaction with alpha adrenoreceptors. *Eur J Pharmacol* 157: 205–213

58 Heilig M, Soderpalm B, Engel JA, Widerlöv E (1989) Centrally administered neuropeptide Y (NPY) produces anxiolytic-like effects in animal anxiety models. *Psychopharmacology* 98: 524–529

59 Heilig M, Koob GF, Ekman R, Britton KT (1994) Corticotropin-releasing factor and neuropeptide Y: role in emotional integration. *Trends Neurosci* 17: 80–85

60 Heilig M, Widerlöv E (1990) Neuropeptide Y: an overview of central distribution, functional aspects, and possible involvement in neuropsychiatric illnesses. *Acta Psychiat Scand* 82: 95–114

61 Kaye WH, Berrettini W, Gwirtsman H, George DT (1990) Altered cerebrospinal fluid neuropeptide Y and peptide YY immunoreactivity in anorexia and bulimia nervosa. *Arch Gen Psychiat* 47: 548–546

62 Widerlöv E, Lindstrom LH, Wahlestedt C, Ekman R (1988) Neuropeptide Y and peptide YY as possible cerebrospinal fluid markers for major depression and schizophrenia. *J Psychiat Res* 22: 69–79

63 Widdowson PS, Ordway GA, Halaws AE (1992) *J Neurochem* 59: 73–80

64 Hedner T, Edgar B, Edvinsson L, Hedner J, Persson B, Petterson A (1992) Yohimbine pharmacokinetics and interaction with the sympathetic nervous system in normal volunteers. *Eur J Clin*

Pharmacol 43: 651–666

65 Boulenger JP, Jerabek I, Jolicoeur FB, Lavallee YJ, Leduc R, Cadieux A (1996) Elevated plasma levels of neuropeptide Y in patients with panic disorder. *Amer J Psychiat* 153: 114–116

66 Stein MB, Hauger RL, Dhalla KS, Charter MS, Asmundson CJ (1996) Plasma neuropeptide Y in anxiety disorders: findings in panic disorder and social phobia. *Psychiat Res* 59: 183–188

67 Britton KT, Southerland S, Van Uden E, Kirby D, Rivier J, Koob G (1997) Anxiolytic activity of NPY receptor agonists in the conflict test. *Psychopharmacology* 132: 6–13

68 Ehlers CL, Somes C, Lopez A, Kirby D, Rivier JE (1997) Electrophysiological actions of neuropeptide Y and its analogs: new measures for anxiolytic therapy? *Neuropsychopharmacology* 17: 34–43

69 Wahlestedt C (1998) Reward for persistence in substance P research. *Science* 281: 1624–1625

70 Penney JB Jr (1996) Neurochemical neuroanatomy. *In*: BS Fogel, RB Schiffer, SM Rao (eds): *Neuropsychiatry*. Williams and Wilkins, Baltimore, 145–171

71 Otsuka M, Yoshioka K (1993) Neurotransmitter functions of mammalian tachykinins. *Physiol Rev* 73: 229–308

72 Kramer MS, Cutler NR, Feighner J, Shrivastava S, Carman J, Sramek JJ, Reines SA, Liu G, Snavely D, Wyatt-Knowles E et al (1998) Distinct mechanism for antidepressant activity by blockade of central substance P receptors. *Science* 281: 1640–1645

73 Nutt DJ (1998) Substance P antagonists: a new treatment for depression? *Lancet* 352: 1644–1646

74 File SE (1997) Anxiolytic action of a neurokinin 1 receptor antagonist in the social interaction test. *Pharmacol Biochem Behav* 58: 747

75 Khantzian EJ, Treece C (1985) DSM-III psychiatric diagnosis of narcotic addicts: recent findings. *Arch Gen Psychiat* 42: 1067–1071

76 Nutt DJ (1991) Anxiety and its therapy: today and tomorrow. *In*: M Briley, SE File (eds): *New concepts in anxiety*. Pierre Fabre Monograph Series, MacMillan Press, 1–12

77 Rubinow DR, Davis CL, Post RM (1995) Somatostatin in the central nervous system. *In*: FE Bloom, DJ Kupfer (eds): *Psychopharmacology. The fourth generation of progress*. Raven Press, New York, 553–562

78 Altemus M, Pigott T, L'Hereux F, Davis CL, Rubinw DR, Murphy DL, Gold PW (1993) CSF somatostatin in obsessive-compulsive disorder. *Amer J Psychiat* 150: 460–464

79 Vecsei L, Widerlöv E (1988) Brain and CSF somatostatin concentrations in patients with psychiatric or neurological illness: an overview. *Acta Psychiat Scand* 78: 657

80 Kakigi T, Maeda K, Kaneda H, Chihara K (1992) Repeated administration of antidepressant drugs reduces regional somatostatin concentrations in rat brain. *J Affect Disord* 25: 215–220

81 Abelson JL, Nesse RM, Vinik A (1990) Treatment of panic-like attacks with a long-acting analogue of somatostatin. *J Clin Psychopharmacol* 10: 128–132

82 Coplan JD, Trost RC, Owens MJ, Cooper TB, Gorman JM, Nemeroff CB, Rosenblum LA (1998) Cerebrospinal fluid concentrations of somatostatin and biogenic amines in grown primates reared by mothers exposed to manipulated foraging conditions. *Arch Gen Psychiat* 55: 473–477

83 Okuyama S, Sakagawa T, Chaki S, Imagawa Y, Ichiki T, Inagami T (1999) Anxiety-like behaviour in mice lacking the angiotensin II type-2 receptor. *Brain Res* 821: 150–159

84 Walther T, Voigt JP, Fukamizu A, Fink H, Bader M (1999) Learning and anxiety in angiotensin-deficient mice. *Behav Brain Res* 100: 1–4

85 Kaiser FC, Palmer GC, Wallace AV, Carr RD, Fraser-Rae L, Hallam C (1992) Antianxiety properties of the angiotensin II antagonist, DUP 753, in the rat using the elevated plus-maze. *Neuroreport* 3: 922–924

86 Shepherd J, Bill DJ, Dourish CT, Grewal SS, Mc Lenahan A, Stanhope KJ (1996) Effects of the selective angiotensin II receptor antagonists losartan and PD123177 in animal models of anxiety and memory. *Psychopharmacology* 126: 206–218

87 Van de Kar LD, Rittenhouse PA, Li Q, Levy AD (1996) Serotonergic regulation of renin and prolactin secretion. *Behav Brain Res* 73: 203–208

88 Bing O, Möller C, Engel JA, Soderpalm B, Heilig M (1993) Anxiolytic-like action of centrally administered galanin. *Neurosci Lett* 164: 17–20

89 Mason GA, Garbutt JC, Prange AJ Jr (1995) Thyrotropin-Releasing hormone. Focus on basic neurobiology. *In*: FE Bloom, DJ Kupfer (eds): *Psychopharmacology. The fourth generation of progress*. Raven Press, New York, 493–503

90 Humbert T, Pujalte D, Bottai T, Hue B, Pouget R, Petit P (1998) Pilot investigation of thyrotropin-releasing hormone-induced thyrotropin and prolactin release in anxious patients treated with

diazepam. *Clin Neuropharmacol* 21: 80–85

91 Broqua P, Benyassi A, Grouselle D, Arancibia S (1993) Antidepressant/anxiolytic ipsapirone inhibits cold-induced hypothalamic TRH release. *Neuroreport* 4: 1200–1202

92 Stein MB, Uhde TW (1991) Endocrine, cardiovascular, and behavioural effects of intravenous protirelin in patients with panic disorder. *Arch Gen Psychiat* 48: 148–156

93 Tancer ME, Stein MB, Uhde TW (1990) Paradoxical growth-hormone responses to thyrotropin-releasing hormone in panic disorder. *Biol Psychiat* 27: 1227–1230

94 Tancer ME, Stein MB, Gelertner CS, Uhde TW (1990) The hypothalamic-pituitary-thyroid axis in social phobia. *Amer J Psychiat* 147: 929–933

95 Coupland NJ, Bailey JE, Glue P, Nutt DJ (1995) The cardiovascular and subjective effects of thyrotropin releasing hormone (TRH) and a stable analogue, dimethyl proline – TRH, in healthy volunteers. *Brit J Clin Pharmacol* 40: 223–229

96 Reist C, Kauffmann CD, Chicz-Demet A, Chen CC, Demet EM (1995) REM latency, dexamethasone suppression test, and thyroid releasing hormone stimulation test in posttraumatic stress disorder. *Prog Neuropsychopharmacol Biol Psychiat* 19: 433–443

97 Fossey MD, Lydiard RB, Ballenger JC, Laraia MT, Bissette G, Nemeroff CB (1993) Cerebrospinal fluid thyrotropin-releasing hormone concentrations in patients with anxiety disorders. *J Neuropsychiat Clin Neurosci* 5: 335–337

98 Coupland NJ, Malizia AL, Bailey JE, Nutt DJ (1996) Thyrotropin-releasing hormone: a potential comparator for the panicogenic effects of pentagastrin and CCK? *Biol Psychiat* 39: 465–466

99 Marangell LB, George MS, Callahan AM, Ketter TA, Pazzaglia PJ, L'Herrou TA, Leverich GS, Post PM (1997) Effects of intrathecal thyrotropin-releasing hormone (protirelin) in refractory depressed patients. *Arch Gen Psychiat* 54: 214–222

100 Bunevicius R, Matulevicius V (1993) Short-lasting behavioural effects of thyrotropin-releasing hormone in depressed women: results of placebo-controlled study. *Psychoneuroendocrinology* 18: 445–449

101 Rinaman L, Sherman TG, Stricker EM (1995) Vasopressin and oxytocin in the central nervous system. *In*: FE Bloom, DJ Kupfer (eds): *Psychopharmacology. The fourth generation of progress.* Raven Press, New York, 531–542

102 Wotjak CT, Kubota M, Liebsch G, Montkowski A, Holsboer F, Neumann I, Landgraf R (1996) Release of vasopressin within the rat paraventricular nucleus in response to emotional stress: a novel mechanism of regulating adrenocorticotropic hormone secretion? *J Neurosci* 16: 7725–7732

103 Bhattacharya SK, Bhattacharya A, Chakrabarti A (1998) Anxiogenic activity of intraventricularly administered arginine vasopressin in the rat. *Biog Amines* 14: 367–385

104 Liebsch G, Wotjak CT, Landgraf R, Engelman M (1996) Septal vasopressin modulates anxiety-related behaviour in rats. *Neurosci Lett* 217: 101–104

105 Landgraf R, Gerstberger R, Montkowski A, Probst JC, Wotjak CT, Holsboer F, Engelmann M (1995) V1 vasopressin receptor antisense oligodeoxynucleotide into septum reduces vasopressin binding, social discrimination abilities, and anxiety-related behaviour in rats. *J Neurosci* 15: 4250–4258

106 Altemus M, Pigott T, Kalogeras KT, Demitrack M, Dubbert B, Murphy DL, Gold PW (1992) Abnormalities in the regulation of vasopressin and corticotropin releasing factor secretion in obsessive-compulsive disorder. *Arch Gen Psychiat* 49: 9–20

107 Leckman JF, Goodman WK, North WG, Chappell PB, Price LH, Pauls DL, Anderson GM, Riddle MA, Mc Swiggan-Hardin M, McDougle CJ et al (1994) Elevated cerebrospinal fluid levels of oxytocin in obsessive-compulsive disorder. *Arch Gen Psychiat* 51: 782–792

108 Windle RJ, Shanks N, Lightman SL, Ingram CD (1997) Central oxytocin administration reduces stress-induced corticosterone release and anxiety behaviour in rats. *Endocrinology* 138: 2829–2834

109 McCarthy MM (1995) Estrogen modulation of oxytocin and its relation to behaviour. *Adv Exp Med Biol* 395: 235–245

110 Van de Kar LD, Levy AD, Li Q, Brownfield MS (1998) A comparison of the oxytocin and vasopressin responses to the 5-HT1a agonist and potential anxiolytic drug alnespirone (S-20499). *Pharmacol Biochem Behav* 60: 677–683

111 Unvas-Moberg K, Bjorkstrand E, Hillegaart V, Ahlenius S (1999) Oxytocin as a possible mediator of SSRI-induced antidepressant effects. *Psychopharmacology* 142: 95–101

112 Altemus M, Jacobson KR, Debellis M, Kling M, Rubinow DR, Potter WZ, Rapoport JL (1999)

Normal oxytocin and NPY levels in OCD. *Biol Psychiat* 45: 931–933

113 Swedo SE, Leonard HL, Kruesi MJ, Rettew DC, Listwak SJ, Berrettini W, Stipetic M, Hamburger S, Gold PW, Potter WZ et al (1992) Cerebrospinal fluid neurochemistry in children and adolescents with obsessive-compulsive disorder. *Arch Gen Psychiat* 49: 29–36

114 Fuller RW (1996) Mechanisms and functions of serotonin neuronal systems. *Ann N Y Acad Sci* 780: 176–184

Subject index